THE DACHMAN DIET for kids

THE DACHMAN DIET for kids

A Complete Guide to Healthy Weight Loss

KEN DACHMAN

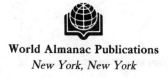

World Almanac Publications
New York, New York

First published in 1986

Distributed in the United States by Ballantine Books, a
division of Random House, Inc., and in Canada by Random
House of Canada, Ltd.

Library of Congress Catalog Card Number 85-51528

Newspaper Enterprise Association ISBN 0-88687-254-5
Ballantine Books ISBN 0-345-33313-6

Printed in the United States of America

World Almanac Publications
Newspaper Enterprise Association
A division of United Media Enterprises
A Scripps Howard company
200 Park Avenue
New York, New York 10166

10 9 8 7 6 5 4 3 2 1

JACKET AND BOOK DESIGN BY BETTY BINNS GRAPHICS

For the many hours of sadness, the years of seemingly boundless frustration, and as repayment for hundreds of dollars in grocery bills, I lovingly dedicate this work to Rhoda and Leonard Dachman, my mom and dad.

And to Uncle Rob, who has always made me proud of my last name. 7102608

CONTENTS

ACKNOWLEDGMENTS

An author is often akin to the general contractor,
whose product is supported by the synthesis of individual
labors. Through their efforts, the following people
helped to lay the foundation on which this work rests:

Lorna M. Castellanos, R.D., an expert in child nutrition,
was extremely helpful with the development of the diet
strategy and companion recipes.

Dr. Susan Swedo's input was essential to establishing and
sustaining a high medical standard for the book.

Beyond his outstanding editorial skills, Daril Bentley
displayed warmth and unbending patience throughout.

Connie Clausen and Guy Kettelhack, two of New York's
finest literary agents, taught me the value of succinct
communication.

Arlene Uslander has always been generous in her support of
my efforts. She encouraged the production of this book
from its very inception.

And special thanks to Pam Liebing, who helped me to "glue"
it all together.

INTRODUCTION

Susan Swedo, M.D., F.A.A.P.
Division Chairwoman, Child and Adolescent Medicine
Evanston Hospital, Chicago

THE *Dachman Diet for Kids* is a thoughtful, well-organized book for parents concerned about their child's obesity. It is difficult to choose a safe, effective diet plan for children and adolescents from the plethora of materials available. *The Dachman Diet for Kids* fulfills all the requirements of a diet book for children; it is medically sound, nutritionally complete, and deliciously effective; add to these the fact that your child will like the foods on his plate and you have a winner!

Personal anecdotes from Ken Dachman provide a window to the heart and mind of an obese child. Through this window, one is able to see the fears of staying fat and the immense obstacles to becoming thin that the child experiences. Thus enlightened, parents are able to sensitively and effectively enable their child to become thin. Of particular importance are the issues of environmental influences and emotional hunger. It is these that parents are able to control. The decision to lose weight must come from the child, however. As Mr. Dachman points out, *he* decided to lose weight and then required his parents' support and assistance to begin and stay with his weight loss program.

The diet plans have been designed in conjunction with a pediatric dietician. At first, it may seem strange to see a diet plan with hot dogs, pork and beans, peanut butter, and cookies, but each of these offers necessary nutrients, and limited portion sizes result in controlled weight loss. The menus are so appetizing that it will be easy for the entire family to "diet" without noticing, much less suffering. As physicians have become more knowledgeable about the benefits of good nutrition and the harm of excess salt, sugar, and fat, we now encourage everyone—whether fat, thin, or just right—to adopt the healthy eating habits outlined in this book.

Exercise is the other important ingredient in the formula of weight loss. Your child must not be forced to exercise, or he will soon hate it, and rebel by becoming even more sedentary. Rather, exercise should become a regular part of the family's and his day. Individual sports are preferred because they can be continued after high school, and a variety of indoor and outdoor activities ensures his year-round participation.

Following the "Dachman Diet" virtually guarantees weight loss for your child. Changed habits, such as exercising, measuring food amounts, and eating only when physically hungry, combined with an improved self-image, ensure maintenance of this loss. Before beginning this plan, as with any weight-loss program, you should check with your child's doctor. As a pediatrician, I highly recommend *The Dachman Diet for Kids.*

THE DACHMAN DIET for kids

1

THE OBESITY NIGHTMARE

I F I had my life to live over again, I would give anything not to have had to go through the torment I experienced as an obese child and teenager. The saddest part is the realization that the torment could have been avoided if my parents had been given the kind of advice and guidance that is available in this book. The information herein is the result of my childhood struggle to lose 250 pounds, and of ten years of fieldwork conducted in weight-loss clinics and in lectures and workshops given across the country.

The Psychological Burden of Obesity

A fat child *is* a sad child, and more often than not, grows up to be a sad adult. The person who first promoted the phrase, "Fat people are jolly," must have been a major stockholder in a cupcake factory. That premise is false—you know it, I know it, and most of all, any fat person knows it.

Society can be unbelievably cruel to overweight people. It seems that when one is extremely overweight, he or she is often automatically classified as some sort of aberration—a freak of nature. This cruel typecasting is especially difficult for children to understand and to deal with, because youngsters have not had time to develop the coping mechanisms that many overweight adults learn as they mature.

The overweight child bears a tremendous psychological and social burden. But how does it *really feel* to be a fat child? The following are just a few of the candid comments children from my weight-loss clinics have shared with me, knowing that I could empathize with them only too well.

Eight-year-old George: "The worst part about being fat is having to go to school. Most of the kids in my class call me 'Hanky the Hippo.' Nobody likes me and I never get to play kickball at recess 'cause the kids say a 'fatso' like me can't run good enough!"

Sixteen-year-old Jenny: "I'm the only girl in my class who wasn't invited to the prom. I told my mother and she said, 'It's your own fault. Maybe if you would lose some weight like I keep telling you to do, the boys would give you a second look.'"

Eighteen-year-old Don: "I've always found it hard to make friends. People always seem to have judged me on how I look, not who I am. So I'm not a real slender guy—so what? I made the Dean's List in college last semester. Doesn't that count for something?"

Ten-year-old Chris: "Nobody ever wants to sit next to me in class. All the other kids write mean notes about how fat I am, and always hold their noses when I walk into the room. I wish I could be Sally English, because she's so thin and pretty; everybody likes her."

Most overweight children subvert the feelings expressed in the foregoing comments and rarely reveal them to anyone, least of all their parents. Your child may not tell you about his negative experiences, but, believe me, they happen every day. The truth is simply too painful to admit, and often he or she just suffers in silence.

At a time in life when he should be discovering his talents, developing an interest in the world around him, growing in self-confidence, and meeting new challenges, the overweight child is at a sad disadvantage. Many (often most) of his peers don't like him; in fact, typically, they will ostracize him because he is "different." Their cruel taunts can destroy his budding self-image before it has a chance to bloom.

Overweight children (and all lonely children, for that matter) will often resort to pitiful tactics in an attempt to transcend their "outcast" status. For example, they use bribery to attract playmates, as I did. I would beg my parents for the latest, most expensive toys on the market, knowing that those toys would bring neighborhood kids to my door—at least until the novelty wore off. I would insist on having an expensive new football, knowing that if I provided the ball, the other boys would be forced to let me play.

Of course, these ploys provide the most fleeting of solutions for an obese child. He often feels inferior, is depressed, and becomes increasingly alienated from his peer group. As a result, many overweight children eventually come to *prefer* a "loner" role as insulation against repeated rejection by others.

School and the Overweight Child

Educational performance can be another misfortune in the life of an overweight child. How can an obese child stand up to recite in class or walk to the blackboard to solve a math problem, knowing he must endure the mocking stares of his classmates. How can he develop a spirit of achievement when he already views himself in a negative light. As a child in one of my classes put it, "What's the use of trying for an 'A'? Nobody really cares anyway."

Even when an overweight child scores higher on intelligence tests than his thinner classmates, his classroom grades will seldom reflect his abilities. Nor will he be drawn to athletic competition or club membership; the risk of rejection is just too great. Many teachers will also admit that it's easy to ignore the quiet overweight student in favor of his more outgoing and attractive classmates.

Adolescence to Adulthood

The teen years are difficult enough for the "normal" child; for the overweight adolescent, they can be devastating. It is often in high school that the overweight teenager's personality solidifies into the tangle of bitterness and self-rejection that will stay with him for the rest of his life. At this stage, he also begins to experience the unspoken social discrimination that will plague his adult years. The overweight adolescent is often left out of the teenage social round of parties, dances, and dating. Studies also suggest that obese high school seniors are less likely to be accepted by colleges than their thinner classmates with the same entrance scores.

As the overweight adolescent reaches adulthood, he will soon discover that his weight problem may adversely affect his career plans. Statistics show that overweight people have a tougher time finding a job, and, once hired, are less likely to be promoted or placed in high-visibility, public-contact positions. One personnel expert estimates that every ten pounds of excess weight costs an aspiring executive $1,000 in annual salary.

The Health of Your Child

It is clear that obesity can cause social and emotional problems, but there is another important reason why we, as parents, must make every effort to help heavy children *become* thin, and to help thin children *remain* thin. That reason is, very simply, good health.

You may have already noticed that your overweight youngster is susceptible to respiratory ailments, anemia, or skin rashes, but, like most parents, you probably think of children as immune to such disorders as hypertension (high blood pressure), cardiovascular disease, and arthritis. The fact is, however, that overweight children tend to show an increased propensity toward such disorders. Furthermore, as overweight children get older, the chance of their being stricken by one or more of these serious diseases is greatly increased.

Within the last ten years, considerable medical research has supported the theory that being overweight increases one's susceptibility to heart disease. Although it is not considered to be a *direct* cause of heart disease, obesity is a serious *indirect* factor. For example, obesity is a contributing factor of hypertension, which, in turn, increases the likelihood of heart attacks.

Because the bodies of overweight youngsters are constantly growing and changing, the effects of obesity on their skeletal systems is also cause for concern. Each of us has protective sac-like organs surrounding our joints, called bursae. The bursae cushion and protect the bone joints against physical trauma. When a child is overweight, his body is forced to carry an extra burden; as a result, the bursae are stretched beyond their natural limits and can eventually deteriorate. When this happens, the bones may start to erode. This condition can gradually lead to bursitis and arthritic ailments.

Aside from these specific ills, there is no question that obesity robs a child of the comfort and general feeling of physical well-being that most other children take for granted. Because of the added strain on his skeleton, and on his respiratory and cardiovascular systems, the overweight youngster is often short of breath after walking a very short distance or after climbing a flight of stairs. He may experience muscular pain, particularly in his back and legs. Most childhood recreation requires energy and activity, but the overweight youngster has limited mobility and is easily fatigued. He is forced to adopt a sedentary lifestyle, which exacerbates his weight problem.

Toward a More Positive Self-Image

It is so important for a child to feel good about himself, to have a positive self-image. How a child perceives himself affects everything he does, present and future. How a child looks plays a big role in this perception, as well. The heavy child seldom feels good about himself, because, as was pointed out earlier, he is different from the "norm," a fact which others bring to his attention all too readily.

Overweight youngsters tend to carry this self-image into adulthood. Because their childhood social relationships were often so difficult, many overweight adults find it hard to develop and sustain emotional attachments. Some restrict their social lives to acquaintances who are also overweight, people who share their problem and don't regard them as freaks.

Of course, not all overweight youngsters have social or emotional problems; some have happy childhoods, supportive families, and many friends, despite the handicap of their obesity, but the simple fact is that *being overweight is never an asset to a child*, either physically or emotionally. Your child can overcome this handicap if you are willing to help him. It will take time, effort, and plenty of love, but the results will be well worth it.

Read *The Dachman Diet for Kids* carefully. Adopt the principles, guidelines, and techniques that have helped thousands of youngsters to lose weight safely. You will not only be helping your child become a happier youngster, but you may be giving him added years of life or, at the very least, healthier, more comfortable years during that life. What greater gift could any parent give a child?

2

MY OWN TRAGEDY—AND TRIUMPH

O N July 29, 1958, a normal seven-pound, seven-ounce baby boy was born in a Chicago hospital, to the delight of his proud parents. By the time the baby was two years old, however, his parents' delight was beginning to turn to concern—even alarm—and their pride was quickly replaced by feelings of embarrassment. You see, the "normal" baby no longer looked quite so normal: he weighed sixty pounds! That sixty-pound two-year-old was *I*.

I kept on gaining weight at a disproportionate rate for my age and height until, at the age of six, I weighed 135 pounds. I was no longer the cute and cuddly fat boy relatives loved to kiss, hug, and pinch, or the adorable, jolly-looking youngster people on the street would smile at and chuck under the chin. At age six, I had become a misfit—a social outcast. Both in the neighborhood and at school, I was the object of teasing and taunting by my peers, and even by unthinking, insensitive adults. The ridicule and ostracism with which I had to contend, on a daily basis, caused me so much emotional pain that I began to dread walking out my front door; I feared that some of the neighborhood kids would be outside waiting to make fun of me. Often, my fears were well-grounded because, sure enough, when I went outside, there they were. Let me share with you an incident that will *never* leave my memory.

I was six years old and watching television after school one afternoon when I heard a great deal of commotion outside. I opened the front door to investigate and saw about a dozen kids marching around my lawn in procession, carrying large, brightly-painted signs. "We Hate You Dachman!" said one sign. "You Sicken Us, You Big Fat Pig!" said another. I don't have to tell you what a traumatic experience that was for a six-year-old.

My family had to change its phone number three times because of abusive calls about my weight problem. The kids would call up and say things to my parents, such as "Is this where Kenny Dachman lives? We're thinking of taking up a neighborhood collection for him. You folks must have awfully big grocery bills!" Or, "Tell Blimpo, the minute he walks out of the house, we're going to stampede him and stomp his fat face into the ground." Sometimes, callers wouldn't even refer to me; they would just shout obscenities into the phone, and we assumed it was my weight problem that provoked the attack.

In a way, I suppose I invited, or at least encouraged, all the teasing, because instead of letting the verbal abuse "go in one ear and out the other," as my parents kept imploring me to do, I soaked it all up. Instead of fighting back and punching one or two of my tormentors (who always weighed considerably *less* than I did), I would lock myself in my bedroom with my radio—my trusty old friend —and cry. That seemed to be my only release from the day's tensions—that and *eating*.

When the kids saw that I retreated, they kept coming back for more "fun and games" at the expense of the "neighborhood blimp," as I came to be called. This behavior, of course, wasn't surprising. Any child with a noticeable problem, be it a physical or social handicap, or a learning disability—any child who is the slightest bit different from the majority of his or her peers, even if "being different" means that his mother makes him wear a yellow raincoat, when all the rest of the kids in his class wear red—is fair game for abuse. The child who refuses to take the abuse, however, having learned to fight back, or having developed enough internal fortitude to ignore it, is the one most likely to escape further abuse. However, the child who takes the taunting and jeering, and then retreats, is usually the one who will be tortured the most—as I was.

By age ten, I weighed 200 pounds. The ridicule became so unbearable that I slowly withdrew from school, having developed a classic case of "school phobia." I made up every excuse I could possibly think of to stay home, and became a master at fooling my mother into thinking I was sick.

Had I put as much effort into my schoolwork as I did into *avoiding* school, I might have been valedictorian of my class. When the excuses didn't work, I often played hooky. On the days when I had no choice but to go to school, because one of my parents would deliver me there in person, I tried my best to keep away from gym class: the thought of being made to participate in sports, at which I was terribly clumsy, made me shudder with fear.

You might think that all the jokes, all the taunts, and all the problems I had to face every day would have been strong enough motivation to make me want to lose weight. On the contrary, the more people made fun of me, the more food I would consume. It was a never-ending, vicious circle.

My parents took me to all kinds of professionals—child psychologists, psychiatrists, weight-loss doctors—and to weight-loss clinics and self-help groups. I was given enough advice, instruction, and diets to fill an encyclopedia, but nothing seemed to work for me—at least, not for more than a few weeks at a time. By the time I reached eighth grade, I was carrying around nearly 280 pounds on my five-foot, five-inch frame, and was as miserable, I believe, as any child could possibly be. I was afraid to talk to people, knowing how repulsive I must have looked in their eyes. When I was forced, out of necessity, to speak to someone other than a family member, I was always on the defensive, preparing myself way ahead of time for the other person's verbal assault. As I mentioned previously, I attended school as little as possible, but when I did go, I couldn't concentrate in class; I didn't listen. Instead, I was off in my own world because I was afraid to be in the *real* world—a world which caused me so much unhappiness. Finally, I stopped going to school altogether.

Survival Tactics

The day after my eighth-grade graduation, I was admitted to what my parents and I had been led to believe was a private residential school, affiliated with a large, highly reputable Chicago hospital. The professionals who had recently made recommendations as to how I could lose weight, and thereby lead a happier, more comfortable life, pointed out that the only way I could possibly achieve that goal would be for me to get away from my family, home environment, and school for an unspecified period of time. My parents welcomed the idea, hoping and praying that the structured program of the "private school," along with the change of environment, would help me to become more comfortable, more responsible, and more importantly, *thinner.*

The "private school" wasn't what my parents or I had expected, however. It turned out that I spent the next sixteen months confined to the psychiatric floor of the hospital where there was a "school program," but where I also learned about a side of life which was as foreign to me as life on another planet. I was only thirteen years old, a very young adolescent who had never even slept away from home. I was suddenly forced not only to be apart from my parents and brothers, but to be part of a world which terrified me night and day.

I will never forget how deceived, trapped, and lonely I felt—as though, somehow, this horrible experience was a direct result of my obesity. I believed I was being punished for being a freak—for being different. I later discovered that, although my parents were also upset about the length of my stay and the nature of the institution itself, they felt compelled to leave me there for "my own good."

When I entered the hospital, I weighed approximately 280 pounds. When I came out, almost a year and a half later, I was fatter than ever, weighing in excess of 400 pounds, which bulged over my sixty-four-inch waist. One of the acute ironies of my hospital stay was that I was never actually put on a diet. As I later found out, however, weight loss was not the primary objective of my therapy program, but rather, getting Kenny Dachman to know more about himself. My therapist left it up to me to record my weight periodically, as part of my "responsibility awareness" training.

Obviously, I wasn't ready to be *that* responsible. When I stepped on the scale and saw the indicator go up to 350 pounds, I would mark 300 on my chart. When the scale wouldn't register any more poundage, I wrote down 340 pounds. I realize now, of course, that I was fooling no one but myself; nevertheless, this was the type of unstructured weight-control treatment I received in the hospital.

When I arrived home from the hospital, many of my former problems still existed. I had few friends; I wasn't able to get dates or strike up relationships with girls. Unable to fit into the stylish clothes I wanted to wear, I had no alternative but to wear the same out-of-date "old men's"-type clothes day after day. I was now fatter than ever, weighing in at 410 pounds. In other words, I still had all of the problems associated with my obesity—problems that were clearly visible. What I didn't realize when I first came out of the hospital was that even though I looked the same, I had undergone a very important change. During my sixteen-month stay in the hospital, I had developed a subliminal strength, a "survivor" mentality which made me feel more assertive.

Once home from the hospital, I spent a year becoming reacclimated to my family and peers. I was much more comfortable with myself than I had been before entering the hospital, and I had a good handle on just who Ken Dachman was. I was also much better able to deal with my problems, past and present. Sure, people still made fun of me, but I started to fight back. Instead of running away when someone jumped on me and hit me, I would hit back (not a response I would endorse, but one that showed my new determination). When someone taunted me verbally, I talked back, instead of retreating into my shell. My new assertive attitude showed an important part of my emotional growth. This attitude would ultimately help me develop and stick to a diet, and become the thin person I had always wanted to be.

Success at Long Last

On New Year's Eve of 1974, my parents gave a big party. There were dozens of trays of food: huge platters of smoked fish and cold cuts; rolls and bread; salads; luscious-looking, rich pastries; and every kind of candy and nuts you can imagine. Normally, on such occasions, I would wait until no one was looking, fill a sack or two with an assortment of food, and run down to the basement or into my bedroom so that I could gorge myself, to my stomach's content, in private bliss. But that night, I just didn't feel like eating as much as I usually did. In fact, for the first time in my life, at age sixteen, the thought of sneaking food actually seemed repulsive to me.

I decided to go down to the basement, because the basement was the only place that seemed safely tucked away from the rest of the scary world. Underground, in the dark, nobody would bother me; nobody could get to me; nobody could *see* me. On that particular night, all I wanted to do was lie down, relax, and listen to some of my favorite songs on the stereo. I couldn't face my relatives, and I wasn't up to hearing the old, familiar comments: "Oh, Kenny, you'd be so handsome if you only lost weight." Or, "Hey, Ken, you'd make a great linebacker if you would turn some of that excess weight into muscle."

Walking downstairs, I passed my older brothers, who were on their way to the party. They were joking with and punching each other in a playful manner, talking about the dates they'd had the weekend before and about possibly going skiing the following weekend. Their conversation was really no different from usual, but on *this* night, it suddenly hit me, like a slap in the face, how completely different their lives were from mine. They weren't that much older than I—only a few years. Why should *they* have all the fun, participate in all the sports they wanted to, have all the dates, I asked myself, when all I did was feel sad, unpopular, and bored most of the time? It just didn't make sense. I knew they cared about me, and I cared about them, but at that moment, I envied them almost to the point of hatred.

A few hours later, after listening to my favorite records at least three times, I decided to go upstairs. I was feeling very sorry for myself, depressed about all the things I was missing in life. Once upstairs, my depression deepened as I listened to my parents and their guests laughing, and I realized that I had nothing to laugh about. Soon, I started to get hungry. I smelled the cold cuts in my mind; I visualized the pastries and candies, and started to crave those foods when, just a short time before, I had been sickened by the sight of them.

I walked past the kitchen and was about to grab a handful of cup-cakes when, instead, I made a slight detour to the pantry where my mother kept her car keys. I took them off the hook, ran outside, opened the door of my mother's car, and got inside. I turned on the radio and just sat there, my big belly squeezed uncomfortably behind the steering wheel. I really didn't know what I was going to do next. Then, sudden-ly, I sat up straight, turned off the radio, and decided I was going to psych myself into getting ready to lose weight. But every time I thought about all the benefits of losing weight, and how much I want-ed to become thin, I reminded myself of all the times I had tried to diet and had failed. In my mind, the failures kept overriding my dreams of success. My desire to lose weight and my anxieties about facing anoth-er failure were in conflict.

The party ended. I went upstairs to my room and fell onto the bed without undressing, hoping that I could fall asleep quickly so I wouldn't have to deal with my inner struggle. But I couldn't get to sleep; all I could do was think about my situation. It occurred to me, for once in my life, that it was absolutely foolish for me to accept my-self as I was, when I really didn't like myself. It was one thing, I told myself, if people had physical abnormalities as the result of a disease, birth defect, or disfiguring accident, but when a person looked as un-sightly as I did, and there was no physiological disorder involved, that person had to do something about it. I *was* going to do something about it. I *had* to!

In the past, when I made the decision to start a diet the following day, the night before was always especially difficult because, fearing failure again, I would also fear waking up in the morning. New Year's Eve, 1974 was no exception. I had horrible nightmares, fearing that I would fail again or, worse, not even start my diet. Those nightmares, of course, were simply mirrored images of my subconscious. Every obese person has a subconscious part of him that fights against the ef-fort he knows it will take to become thin. It is painful to realize that you can't just relax and be "normal" like most of the other people you know, that *you* have to work especially hard to be "normal." As an obese person, you have to make sacrifices and exert all kinds of self-con-trol simply to attain a state that most people take for granted.

That night I dreamt that, after losing fifty pounds, I gave in to a terrible craving for chocolate and ran to my favorite candy shop. Seeing that it was closed, I picked up a large rock and hurled it through the window. Then I reached inside and unlocked the door. Once in the shop, I began to savagely devour every piece of candy in sight. Afterwards, I heard loud snickering and jeers. "Look at that fat pig—he'll never be thin!" someone shouted. "Kenny, the slob, isn't like us," yelled someone else, "he's food crazy!" Anticipating my neurotic binge, all the kids in the neighborhood had followed me to the candy store. There they began to form a circle and close in on me, chanting, "You'll never be thin! You'll never be thin!..."

In the past, this kind of nightmare would have made me forego my diet. This time, however, I could see that the consequences of being fat were so unbearable, so cruel, that the pleasure I would get from continuing to stuff myself with food simply wouldn't be worth it. I stuck to my decision, harnessing all the willpower I could possibly muster, and soon designed a diet program for myself that I thought (and hoped) would work for me. For the first time in my life, I was able to focus on my present needs and future goals, rather than just on my past experiences.

That night, December 31, 1974, was the cornerstone of my permanent weight loss of 250 pounds and thirty-one inches of waistline. I would be less than honest if I told you that, from that point on, it was easy sailing. It wasn't! There were fears, anxieties, traumas, and setbacks during the year and a half that followed. There were even failures, but the failures were short-lived; the willpower and hard work triumphed, and I reached my lifelong dream of becoming thin. Now I carry 190 pounds around on a six-foot frame.

3

WHY IS MY CHILD OVERWEIGHT?

WE'VE all seen the skinny kid (or adult) who consumes lumber-jack meals every few hours and never gains an ounce. Then there's *your* youngster, who seems to add a pound every time he passes the refrigerator. Why does obesity "happen" to some people and not to others? Is the tendency to be overweight inborn, an inherited trait, or does obesity stem mainly from one's environment?

It is not my purpose here to launch an in-depth investigation into the causes of obesity or to consider the relative merits of various theories. I am more concerned with the cure. It's important to understand what you're up against when battling childhood obesity. Several decades of research have produced valuable insights into this subject, and we should look at the relevant points.

Before we do, however, there's one thing you should know. Obesity is *not* the result of some moral weakness or character flaw. There are a number of physiological and psychological reasons for obesity. When many thin people see an obese person, they often ask themselves, why doesn't he lose weight? Doesn't he *want* to be thin? Doesn't he have any self-respect?

Fat people are no more weak-minded or weak-willed (in areas

other than weight loss) than anyone else. They do struggle for self-respect. It just so happens that their particular problem centers on food, and an inability to say no when they don't really need it. All overweight people—and that includes your child—truly *want* to be thin. For some *legitimate* reason, however, whether physical or behavioral, they cannot achieve that goal. The good news is that, despite these factors, and with your help, your child can break his unhappy eating pattern and find more productive ways of handling his life.

Before you and your child can work to overcome his obesity, you need to understand the causes. Are obese children born or made? Let's look at the facts.

Physiological Factors: Is Obesity Inborn?

Breeders have built fortunes by recognizing that certain kinds of livestock gain and retain weight more easily than others. This is a physical trait, apparently passed on from generation to generation. Some medical experts believe that the tendency to gain and retain weight is a trait inherited by humans as well. As support for their position, these experts point to the fact that overweight parents tend to have overweight kids. Statistics tell us that when both parents are obese, eight out of ten of their children grow up obese. When one parent is obese and the other is of normal weight, that number drops to four out of ten. When both parents are of normal weight, less than one in ten children grows up overweight.

Probably the most talked-about physiological contributors to obesity are *glandular disorders*, such as hypoactive thyroid. These conditions are rare, however. Only one in ten thousand cases of obesity can be directly traced to glandular disorders.

Researchers have recently discovered another possible contributor to obesity, a problem with the body's sensations of hunger and satiety, or "fullness." The *appestat* (a combination of the words "appetite" and "thermostat") is the name for the mechanism in the brain which regulates—turns "on" and "off"—our desire to eat. Nutritionist

Norman Joliffe has found that the appestat is more sensitive in obese people than in thin people. This means that overweight people feel hungry more often than people of normal weight.

Body type is another physiological factor which seems to affect weight. There is evidence that some body structures tend to accumulate excess pounds more easily than others. Ectomorphs (people who have a tall and slender build) tend to stay slim no matter what they eat. Mesomorphs are muscular and sturdy (many athletes fit into this category), but not necessarily fat. Endomorphs are soft and round, and seem the most prone to obesity.

Similarly, the *set-point theory* suggests that different bodies are "programmed" to weigh different amounts, and that the body's tendency to retain fat is indeed an inherited trait—a kind of physiological fate. Dr. William Bennett, author of *The Dieter's Dilemma* (Basic Books, 1982), writes:

> Each body 'wants' a characteristic quantity of fat and proceeds to balance food intake, physical activity, and metabolic efficiency in order to maintain that amount.

When an overweight person hears that his body is preprogrammed for a certain weight, he may (understandably) adopt a "why bother?" attitude. For example, I used to believe I would always be fat, that nothing I did or didn't do would make any difference. It took me a long time to realize that, even though the biological odds might be tipped against me, I *could* lose weight and keep it off.

Environmental Factors: Is Obesity Created?

We've already seen that overweight parents tend to have overweight children. But is this tendency *always* the result of heredity, or is it possible that overweight parents (and sometimes parents of normal weight) create an environment of obesity which causes their kids to become fat and stay fat? Many experts now believe that, in most cases, a child's environment is the strongest influence on his weight.

As an example of the influence of environment, consider the "fat household syndrome." An overweight mom and dad may indeed have overweight offspring, but they're also likely to have fat adopted children, fat dogs, fat hamsters, and canaries that look like tennis balls. Why? Because overeating is the norm in these households. But "fat households" don't misuse food purely out of ignorance or carelessness. There's often a purpose behind the bad eating habits: food can be used to solve problems and accomplish objectives. It can be used as a reward or a punishment, for example: "If you behave in the supermarket, Mamma will buy you a candy bar" or, "You've been naughty—no dessert for a week."

Food can also be used to express that most sought-after of all emotions—love. Some parents, overweight or not, sincerely regard excess calories and a vast array of goodies as proof of love for their family, but this is an attitude of convenience. Food is always easier to dispense than some of the more complex forms of parental affection and concern. After all, earning the money to buy food, and taking the time to prepare it mean your parents care about you, right?

A child quickly learns to eat for the wrong reasons in a home where food is used to reward, bribe, punish, appease, or celebrate; it is also used or as a substitute for parental discipline, warmth and interest. The family strategy teaches a child not to eat because he's hungry, but because he's happy or miserable, proud or fearful. In short, food becomes connected with the kinds of values which have nothing to do with physical hunger or good nutrition.

A family that is raising an overweight child will often substitute food for many of the child's other needs. As soon as the baby starts to fuss, the parents feed him. They rarely stop to determine whether the baby is actually hungry or just cranky. The baby might need cuddling, or a diaper change. He might be too hot or too cold. He might be bored and need a toy, a game of peek-a-boo, or just a few moments of interaction with an understanding adult. In certain families, one kind of attention is usually administered—food. Babies raised in such families, however, soon learn to accept food as the appropriate response to all their needs. In such an environment, eating becomes the major source of emotional comfort for the child.

Let's face it; eating is meant to be an enjoyable experience for everyone, fat or thin. Nevertheless, if food becomes *the* most important part of the family's life, children will attach more significance to it than it deserves. This attachment constitutes what I consider to be the fundamental cause of overeating: *emotional hunger.*

Emotional Hunger

Emotional hunger is the name I assign to food cravings brought about by emotional cues rather than by nutritional needs. It is hunger a person *experiences* physically, but the key to conquering the physical manifestation of hunger is realizing that one is fighting a psychological source in addition to a biological source of that hunger—a hunger which results from feelings of depression, anxiety, loneliness, or even from habit.

Obese people arrive at their condition by eating far beyond their bodily requirement. In fact, they sometimes eat to the point of considerable physical discomfort. Obviously, they are not responding to physical hunger alone, because physical hunger is quickly and easily satisfied, and stops before a point of discomfort is reached. Because emotional hunger *feels* so real, it can overpower the physical sensations that normally signal us to stop eating. The obese among us are eating to make themselves feel better emotionally. Emotions are a very powerful motivator, and emotional hunger, even though it is irrational and often has disastrous consequences, is difficult to overcome.

For example, as a child, I certainly didn't want to be fat, but invariably, after being made fun of by other kids because of my weight, I'd go up to my room, cry awhile, then sneak down to the pantry and grab all the sweets I could find. For me, food was a temporary means of pacifying feelings of rejection, as it is for most overweight children. Even *I* thought my behavior was strange; I knew that by stuffing myself I was only adding to my problems, but I couldn't control myself.

Emotional Hunger Versus Physical Hunger

While emotional hunger is something we *learn*, physical hunger is a natural, instinctive response. To illustrate, consider the dog in the wild. Any naturalist will tell you that a wild dog kills and eats prey only when it is physically hungry. After the dog's appetite has been satisfied, it may not hunt again for several days. Nature has programmed the dog genetically to eat only the amount of food it needs to survive.

Conversely, consider what happens if the dog is domesticated. Suppose it becomes part of a household where it is tossed goodies from the dinner table (even if the dog has just finished a bowl of dog food) and rewarded with a tidbit every time it rolls over or "speaks." Soon, the dog is whining for treats and gaining weight, its natural feeding instinct confused by emotional hunger.

Overweight people manifest this same confusion. They do so much emotional eating that they lose sight of what physical hunger feels like. A leading proponent of the emotional hunger or "externality" theory of overeating is Stanley Schachter, Ph.D., of Columbia University, an authority on obesity. Dr. Schachter conducted several experiments to illustrate that eating can often have little to do with hunger. In one of his experiments, he's shone bright lights on food to make it appear more attractive. Presented with this artificially bright food, obese people ate more than usual. Those taking part in the experiment who were not obese ate their usual amount.

This experiment suggests two conclusions: firstly, the obese person, in particular, is motivated to eat by factors other than hunger; secondly, there seems to be a wide difference between the obese and the nonobese in their psychological attachment to food and in the importance they place on food.

Once a person learns to rely on eating as a way of coping with emotions, it's only a short step to food's becoming a major source of pleasure. Because obese people often feel they have few other sources of emotional gratification, they are resistant to giving up the only source that is really available—food. People who are overweight subconsciously believe that if they don't eat, they will be missing an opportunity to feel good. That's another reason why an obese person will continue to eat past the point at which his appetite has been physically satisfied.

Because emotional hunger is fundamentally different from physical hunger, the foods people eat in order to satisfy an emotional need differ considerably from the kind of food needed for true nutrition. This is particularly unfortunate for those who retain weight easily. Usually, emotional eaters head for the calories—cake, ice cream, potato chips, pastries, and the like. When we're physically hungry, almost any food is appealing to us, but baked fish and carrot sticks just don't do the job when it comes to soothing a broken heart.

Common Sense About Emotional Hunger

There's nothing wrong, of course, with yielding to an occasional spell of emotional hunger. Everyone has a favorite "comfort food" to turn to after a particularly trying day—a bowl of cereal that takes us briefly back to childhood, a cup of cocoa, or a piece of cinnamon toast like Mom used to make for us when we were frightened, cold, or tired.

Emotional eating also has a legitimate social function. It helps to draw people together and it facilitates pleasant relations between strangers, family members, friends, relatives, and business associates. "Breaking bread together" was a venerable human tradition even before biblical times, and feasts shared by early humans celebrating a successful hunt survive, as evidenced by today's lavish dinner parties and business lunches. Nobody would suggest that sensible eating means giving up these occasional bouts of emotionally-gratifying eating and drinking.

However, chronic overeaters cannot confine their emotional eating to these occasional episodes in which physical and emotional hunger are gratified together. They have to do it all the time because they're caught in a vicious circle: they're overweight because they've been using food to quell anixety, and they grow more anxious because they know they are overweight. As a result, they gain more weight, become more upset, and find themselves trapped in a self-defeating ritual that seems to repeat itself endlessly.

It's important to remember, however, that "emotional hunger" is a *learned* response, and what is learned can be *unlearned*. In Chapter 5, "Answers To Dieting Questions," you'll find a simple, but valuable strategy for dealing with emotional hunger and the overeating which accompanies it.

Caution: The American Lifestyle May Be Hazardous To Your Child's Health

Unfortunately, our American lifestyle tends to aid and abet the development of obesity in children. Families rarely sit down together each evening to a well-balanced meal and leisurely conversation. Parents, off on the 7:40 A.M. train, are a missing ingredient in many morning kitchens as well, leaving kids to gulp down sugar-coated cereals or skip breakfast entirely. Lunch in a typical high school cafeteria is often a can of soda and a few bags of potato chips. Too many balanced meals are replaced by less nutritious fast-foods inhaled on the run. Salads? Forget 'em. There's no time to make them. When Americans do find a moment to sit down and relax, it's usually in front of a television set, which opens up a whole new set of opportunities for emotional hunger. Each year the average American child views 21,000 television commercials, half of which are selling junk food. These commercials convey the message that your child will feel great if he eats the advertised product. However, the pleasure is short-lived, and the negative effects are often not worth it.

I hope this chapter has given you a better understanding of the causes of obesity. Whether your child's weight problem arises from an inherited tendency, a legitimate medical condition, or an environment which encourages obesity, *your overweight child can become a thinner, healthier child.* If strong obstacles abound, the struggle may be harder or may take a little longer than expected, but *all* children can lose excess weight and learn to live as healthy people do. I'm living proof that it can be done.

4

HOW TO HELP YOUR CHILD
HELP HIMSELF

Caloriphobia: the Fear of Dieting

A MAJOR reason that so many overweight children have trouble starting or staying on a diet is a fear of perpetual dieting, something I call *caloriphobia*. As I have discussed, food is a major source of pleasure for many people, particularly for children. Your child wants to be thin, but he dreads the idea that he will have to deprive himself of something he really loves in order to reach that goal.

Most overweight children fear that, in order to become thin, they will *never* be able to stop dieting. They will never again be able to eat cookies, or pizza, or doughnuts, or ice cream. What's worse is that this sacrifice seems to be theirs alone. All during my obese childhood, I watched my thin classmates eat the foods they liked, with no obvious ill effects. I envied them because I was convinced that, to be thin like they were, I would have to undergo the incessant torture of dieting. I believed I would never be able to eat the things I liked again.

The overweight child looks at himself in the mirror and sees what a distant goal thinness is. It's very difficult for a child to give up something pleasant *now* in return for something pleasant later. Child development experts tell us that children only gradually learn to forego immediate gratification in order to achieve long-term rewards.

For these reasons, it is painful and traumatic for a child to begin a diet. In fact, it is common for obese children to have nightmares the night before beginning a weight-loss program, as I did. It's much like the night before a battle for a soldier, only your child feels that *this* battle will be unending. He is extremely fearful that he won't be equal to the effort, fearful that he will be miserable in the attempt.

It is vitally important for you as a parent to understand what courage it takes for your child to start a diet program and to stay with it. You can help him overcome his fears about embarking on *this* weight-loss program by sharing several secrets with him.

How to Help Your Child Combat Caloriphobia

First, assure your child that he is not as different from his thin friends as he thinks. Give him a little pep talk that goes something like this: "You have the ability to be thin, too. You just need to learn some things about eating that your friends already know." For example, I eventually realized that my friends who were not overweight could indulge in pizza and ice cream without getting fat because they didn't eat these foods every day. They also ate these foods in moderate amounts. (In Chapter 6, "Your Newly-Thin Child," you will learn more about teaching your child "thin person" behavior.)

You can also let your child in on another secret: the Dachman Diet has been specially designed to combat caloriphobia. Your youngster won't have to diet forever; he will be able to eat his favorite foods even while he is losing weight. *Every day* of the diet program he may spend 300 to 500 bonus calories on "fun" foods which he chooses himself; foods he really enjoys. These can include such favorites as cookies, sweet rolls, milkshakes, and hamburgers. In addition, many foods that kids typically enjoy, such as chocolate milk, spaghetti, and pizza are worked into the diet's meals themselves.

Another Stumbling Block: Desperate Love

Another major obstacle to successful weight loss for children comes from an unexpected quarter—their parents. You probably would never suspect that your well-meant efforts to change the behavior of your overweight child could virtually *assure* that he will continue to gain weight. After all, your actions are honestly motivated by love and concern for your child. This is a phenomenon which I call "desperate love."

Youngsters who attend my weight-loss clinics often talk about their parents' efforts to help them lose weight. One girl found a sign pasted on the refrigerator that proclaimed, "Minutes on the lips, months on the hips." A teenager told me how he came home from school one day to find his posters of rock singers emblazoned with "Fat's not where it's at." The father of a ten-year-old offered her ten dollars for every pound she could lose.

Sometimes these attempts take crueler forms. Parents try to shame their children into losing weight with comments like, "You embarrass me," or "Will you please stop eating? You're disgusting!" Or they take the rest of the family on a trip or to a restaurant, leaving their obese child at home.

Most parents who try to change their children in this way have the best of intentions. They truly love their children and want more than anything for their offspring to be happy and successful. Out of this "desperate love," a parent will go to almost any length to push a child to get better grades, to be more popular, to look more attractive, and, of course, to lose weight. However, because of this kind of concern, a child comes to believe that if his parents are going to such great lengths to change him, they must not love him the way he is. Hurt and angry, the youngster thinks, "Well, if I'm so unloveable, I'll show *them*." In the case of the overweight child, this rebellious attitude (whether conscious or not) takes the form of overeating.

A youngster is likely to suffer through severe bouts of emotional hunger as a result of his parents' desperate love. A child derives his self-image from the world around him: if his parents don't seem to like him the way he is, how can he like himself. As his self-esteem drops, he becomes depressed and eats to comfort himself. He then gains more weight, brings more family pressure upon himself, and feels more depressed. The vicious circle of overeating is complete.

Perhaps I can illustrate the overweight child's response to desperate love through my own example. My parents desperately wanted me to lose weight, and tried every tactic they could think of to help me do so. I remember coming home from school one day to find the kitchen cupboards stripped bare; only a box of baking soda remained. My thin father and brothers would often eat their rich desserts in the bathroom or only after I left the house, to keep me from temptation. At one point, my parents even installed a lock on the refrigerator to prevent my nocturnal raids.

These efforts didn't make me feel loved; instead, I felt pressured to lose weight, "different" because I apparently couldn't be treated like others, and angry because the only attention I received from *anyone* seemed to stem from my size. As a result, I ate even more—partly out of emotional hunger, to comfort myself, and partly to lash back at my parents for making me feel so alien.

How to Conquer Desperate Love

Your youngster needs your support, not desperate attempts to "make" him change. You can break the pattern of desperate love by following these suggestions:

Let your child know you love him, no matter what. It is a great comfort for a child to know that he can be himself, that he can try to work out his problems, even fail, without risking the love of the people who mean the most to him—his parents.

Don't make an issue of your child's weight problem. Instead, try to make a point of recognizing his good qualities: school achievement, special talents, positive personality traits. Take an interest in what he does well. Youngsters need a *balanced* picture of themselves if they are to develop healthy emotional lives.

It is natural to celebrate your child's victories—to buy a new outfit in a smaller size when he loses weight, or to take a special trip to the zoo or the park, but try not to make external rewards the entire goal of your youngster's weight loss. If you bribe your child into losing weight with toys, money, or a trip to Disneyland, he will be dieting for the wrong reasons. The natural consequence of a weight-loss program is *thinness,* with all of its physical and social benefits. Believe me, that is reward enough!

Finally, it must be *your child's* decision to begin a weight-loss program. To become a thin person for life, your child will have to work hard and change many of his old habits. *He must desire to become thin not for you, or for his peers, but for* himself.

Deciding to Diet: Icebreaker Ideas

Now that you know how important it is for your child to begin a weight-loss program on the right emotional footing, here are some tips for breaking the ice.

For Young Children. If your child is between the ages of two and eight, he must rely on *you* to start him on a weight-loss program. However, it is important to make your child feel that weight loss is his goal, too. You might enlist your preschooler's cooperation by suggesting benefits he can easily understand:

"It would really be fun to be able to run fast, wouldn't it?" Working with children in my clinics, I had great success using physical incentives: "When you lose weight, you'll be as strong as He-Man, as fast as Flash, and as agile as Spider Man." Children understand the physical nature of weight loss; the emotional ramifications are usually too abstract for most young minds to grasp. A variation for a slightly older school-age youngster might be: "It would be nice if you could wear those clothes you saw in the store the other day." Or, "You probably would like it if the other children didn't tease you." Then simply say, "Since I love you, I want you to try to lose weight so that these nice things will happen."

For Older Children. Your older child or teen has probably expressed a desire to lose weight already. However, if he hasn't brought up the subject recently, simply open the door for him: "If you ever want to talk about losing weight, let me know. I'd be glad to help you in any way I can." This approach lets your youngster know you care about his problems, and that you are available to help.

If he still shows no interest, wait a month or two, or until he does bring up the subject. Then you might say, "I just bought a book that was written by a guy who was really overweight as a child, but managed to become thin. He seems to have some good ideas and he has helped a lot of kids in his diet clinics lose weight. Would you like to give his program a try?" Because of your truly loving concern, as well as your gentle efforts to promote a weight-loss program, your child can only feel that his decision to diet is a positive one.

5

ANSWERS TO DIETING QUESTIONS

I N the course of conducting weight-loss clinics across the country, I have been asked hundreds of questions about dieting by parents of overweight children. I will address many of these questions in an attempt to anticipate concerns you may have before your child embarks upon the Dachman Diet.

> Our child has tried to lose weight and failed so many times before. How can we expect *this* diet to succeed?

The Dachman Diet has been developed especially for children. The program is not extremely restrictive, nor is it a "fad" diet. It provides enough calories so that your child should never be hungry, and includes a wide variety of menus and recipes selected to suit the tastes of children. This program also offers a great deal of information about the psychological aspects of obesity. Many weight-loss programs fail because they treat the symptoms, while ignoring the causes of overeating. They fail to consider the *whole* child. Your child not only needs to change the way he eats, he also must learn to change the way he *thinks*. (Review Chapter 4, "How To Help Your Child Help Himself.")

Is there a "best time" to begin a diet? My child has expressed a desire to lose weight, but I am concerned about having him begin his diet just before the holidays, when he might be tempted by the many occasions for eating rich foods

Mondays are good days to start diets; the first day of a new week seems like the appropriate time to begin a new life. Holidays pose no threat to dieting success because the Dachman Diet allows your child to eat virtually anything—*in controlled amounts.*

Does my child need a doctor's permission before starting the diet program?

It is always a good idea to consult a physician before making any fundamental change in your child's diet or level of activity. Because the Dachman Diet is nutritionally balanced and medically approved, I see no reason why your doctor would find it unacceptable for your child.

As an obese parent, I feel like a hypocrite encouraging my daughter to follow a diet. How can I expect her to become thin when I can't do it myself?

Of course, the best thing you could do is to diet *with* your child. However, if you can't make the decision to diet, don't let that hold your child back. Explain to your child that you have developed poor eating habits over the years which are very hard to break, and that you don't want her to develop these same habits. You can tell your child that you plan to use all of your energy to help *her* to become thin.

How often should my child weigh himself?

Your child should weigh himself first thing in the morning, twice a week. Regular weigh-ins allow you to monitor your child's progress so that you can make adjustments to his diet if necessary. Weigh-ins also help your child to feel a sense of accomplishment when the scale shows the result of his efforts. However, if your child is losing weight slowly, weigh once a week instead, so that he will not be discouraged about what may appear to be a lack of progress.

What should I tell my child when he complains that other kids can eat anything they want to while he can't?

It's not unusual for a child to feel resentful when he is deprived of the opportunity to eat as he wishes, while those around him aren't similarly deprived. However, don't take his complaint lightly; these feelings of resentment are a major reason for diet failure. (See my comments on *caloriphobia* in Chapter 4, "How To Help Your Child Help Himself".) Tell your child that he will not have to diet forever, that once he reaches his weight goal, he will be able to eat as other people do. You might also mention that nonobese people don't really eat as much as they want all the time, even though it may appear so (see Chapter 6, "Your Newly-Thin Child").

If my child is following the Dachman Diet's 14-Day Menu Plan and does not care for a certain meal, may I substitute a different meal?

Certainly, as long as you substitute a meal from the same level of the diet. For example, a dinner from Day 1 of Plan A may be replaced by a dinner from Day 4 of Plan A. However, do not substitute a lunch for a dinner, or use a meal from another level, because the number and type of servings will not be equivalent. (See Chapter 7, "Getting Started On The Diet" and Chapter 8, "The Dachman Diet," for further information on the Dachman Diet menu plans.)

My child is losing weight rapidly—between five and eight pounds per week—and he complains that he's always hungry. Is this to be expected?

The Dachman Diet is designed to produce a slow, steady weight loss and has sufficient calories to satisfy most appetites. Some initial feelings of hunger are natural, however, as your child adjusts to a reduced caloric intake. If this hunger persists, or if your child is losing weight too rapidly, have him follow the next higher level of the diet (for example, if he's currently following Plan A, start him on Plan B).

Our child is the only one in the family who needs to diet. What can we do to show our support and help him to succeed?

I don't advocate having the entire family change its lifestyle and eating habits to accommodate a child who is dieting; that is simply not realistic. However, you can make dieting easier for your child in a number of ways.

First, you can set a good example by keeping nutritious foods in the house. Make it clear that it's okay to eat "junk food" once in a while, but limit the presence of high-calorie snack foods. This practice will benefit the whole family. You may also find it convenient to serve the dishes from the 14-day menu plans to the entire family. These meals do not differ in any way from normal fare: the recipes and menus provide nutritious, tasty foods that any person will enjoy, whether he's dieting or not. Family members who are not dieting can simply eat larger portions.

Siblings can play an important part—both positive and negative—in a child's weight-loss efforts. Explain to other children in the family that dieting is difficult, and that their support and encouragement can help. Ask them not to tease the dieting youngster with the fact that they can eat things he can't. However, if a sibling won't cooperate willingly, don't force the issue. If you do, the dieting child will be tormented even more—only behind your back. If these problems do occur, let your dieting child know that you are aware of what's going on and that you feel it is unkind. Remind him not to let others stand in the way of his success. You might also suggest that ignoring the behavior of his siblings is probably the best way to eliminate the teasing.

Family members should let the dieting child know they notice his progress, but be careful not to go overboard, shouting, "Wow, I can't believe you've lost weight!," and don't comment on the weight loss ten times a day. It is also quite important to let your child know you are proud of him, that you know dieting isn't easy and takes great willpower. This lets the child know you are focusing on his inner strengths rather than outward appearance. Don't give left-handed compliments which put pressure on your child, or imply that you were horrified with him before he began to lose weight with comments like, "Thank God you're losing weight; I never thought you'd be able to do it!" It's better to make no comment than to pay him that kind of compliment.

My child has had bouts with diarrhea since starting the Diet. Should I be concerned?

The Dachman Diet is a balanced program and should not cause your child to develop any uncomfortable physical symptoms. However, any drastic change in one's diet can cause temporary problems, such as diarrhea, constipation, or even fatigue as the body adjusts to a new regimen. If these problems persist, consult your physician.

Is it all right for us to let our youngster cheat once in a while and eat something she has a real taste for?

Don't undermine your child's efforts by allowing her to go off her diet. The Dachman Diet offers sufficient calories and variety so that your child need never be hungry or bored with the program. Additionally, if there is some specific food your child desires, she can use her "bonus calories," which allow her to satisfy an occasional craving without giving up the discipline of the Diet. She will learn that she can eat her favorite foods without having to "cheat." (See page 75 for more information on using bonus calories.)

Can exercise help my child lose weight faster?

Yes, it can. The simple fact is that we take in calories by eating, and we burn calories through activity. Those calories which are not metabolized become excess fat. If your child increases his level of activity, he is likely to lose weight faster. In addition to burning calories, regular exercise helps to tone up flabby skin, and tends to decrease one's appetite. Regular, strenuous workouts tend to raise the body's level of glucose, serotonin, noradrenaline, adrenaline, and dopamine. Scientists believe that all of these substances inhibit hunger.

Let me make it clear that it is *not* necessary for your child to engage in a regimented program of exercise—daily calisthenics, for example. Dieters often find a strict exercise regimen difficult to adhere to because they are already giving so much mental energy and willpower to the diet itself. Overburdening your child in this way can lead to diet failure.

If you think that it is important for your child to make regular exercise a part of his life, let him ease into an active life gradually. Begin with nonthreatening activities like walking or bicycling, and involve the entire family. If your child is truly unwilling, or rusty from months or years of inactivity, disguise the exercise in the form of a trip to the zoo or the park. Exercise your child truly enjoys won't be seen as a chore.

Our son has little time for breakfast before he catches the bus for school. Can he skip breakfast and add those portions to his lunch?

No! Breakfast is unquestionably the day's most important meal; it provides energy for your child's school activities and promotes alertness. Eating a good breakfast can also keep your child from feeling so hungry that he overindulges later in the day.

In general, encourage your child not to "save" calories during the day in order to gorge himself at one meal, but rather to eat all meals and snacks in the designated portions, and at regular intervals. Studies have shown that eating a number of smaller, more frequent meals can add up to more weight loss than consuming the same number of calories in fewer meals. Our bodies seem to burn calories more efficiently when those calories are consumed gradually. Your child can reinforce the habit of eating only at the specified times by brushing his teeth immediately after each meal and snacktime. Doing so will give him a clean, fresh feeling, and signal that eating time is over.

My child really enjoys diet drinks, but I've heard that they are not healthful. Should she continue to drink diet soda?

Diet sodas can be very satisfying to a dieting child with a sweet tooth. For this reason, diet sodas are included in the 14-day menu plans and in several of the Dachman Diet recipes. I would recommend, however, that you use decaffeinated sodas, and use them only in moderation. Diet sodas (and many other diet products) generally contain either aspartame or saccharin. You can make an intelligent choice between these products if you understand how they differ.

Aspartame, commonly known as NutraSweet, is a compound of two amino acids, phenylalanine and aspartic acid. Amino acids are the substances used to build protein and are found quite naturally in the human body and in most foods—especially milk, meat, eggs, and cheese. Like all amino acids, aspartame is digested and absorbed into the body, and does provide calories. However, because it is 180 times sweeter (more potent) than sugar, only extremely small amounts are required to sweeten beverages and other foods.

Aspartame has been evaluated for safety in more than one hundred studies over a period of eighteen years and has been approved by the Food and Drug Administration. In addition, the American Diabetic Association has recently approved its use for diabetics. Most physicians don't restrict the use of aspartame, but suggest that it be used in moderation.

Saccharin is not absorbed by the body, and thus provides no calories. Because its safety has been questioned by health professionals, you should discuss the use of saccharin with your doctor. Generally, most physicians suggest a limit of two or three servings a day. (A single serving would consist of one can of most diet sodas, or a one-serving packet.)

If you choose to limit your child's consumption of diet soda, you will find a number of good beverage alternatives in the recipe section.

What should I do if my child is not losing weight on the Diet?

Children who are only slightly overweight may not lose weight quickly. Also, keep in mind that children grow rapidly; by not *gaining* weight, your child may actually be growing into his or her proper weight range. If your child is considerably overweight and not losing pounds even though he is adhering to the diet, switch to the next lower level. (You may want to consult your doctor before doing so.) For example, if your child is currently following Plan B, switch to Plan A. If your youngster is already on Plan A, you may reduce the number of bonus calories. However, do not cut your child's daily calorie intake to less than Plan A allows without your doctor's consent.

> How can we prevent our child from overeating when he's angry, lonely, or bored? He truly wants to lose weight, but there are times when he just can't seem to control the urge to overeat.

Your child is responding to emotional hunger, which, as you may recall from Chapter 3, "Why Is My Child Overweight?", is the primary cause of overeating. Most people who are overweight *do* realize when they're overeating. They have a very real understanding that they're doing themselves harm or risking the success of their diet, but at the time, the momentary pleasure of eating is more important than the negative consequences of doing so.

The strategy I have devised to combat emotional hunger makes it impossible to ignore the consequences of overeating. I call this exercise the "ABC's": *Action Before Consequences.* The ABC's are questions your child should always ask himself when he is about to eat something beyond the requirements of the diet, or when he *feels* he shouldn't be eating. These questions are designed to make your child consider the consequences of his actions.

Think about the *action* you are about to take:

> What kind of food am I about to eat? (If your child is craving calorie-laden foods, especially sweets, he should consider this to be a strong sign of emotional hunger.)

Think about the *consequences*:

> If I overeat, will I feel better or worse? (This question forces your child to think about the consequences of overeating before-

hand, rather than become horribly depressed and guilty afterward, when the damage has already been done.)

Right now, what is more important to me, losing weight or giving in? (In other words, are the long-term consequences worth the short-term gratification?)

Encourage your child to *write out* the answers to these questions. If the situation doesn't allow for this, have him answer the questions verbally or mentally.

At first, it may be difficult for your child to do the ABC's; after all, it is far easier to block out negative feelings and experience the pleasure of eating than it is to grapple with the unpleasant consequences. For an overweight child, emotional eating is almost a reflexive behavior. Pausing on the brink of overeating requires tremendous willpower. However, after the first few times your child uses the ABC's to withstand the temptation to overeat, he will feel good about himself; he will experience a sense of control over his own behavior. As he begins to lose weight, he will have proof that overeating is a transitory pleasure at best, while being thin has innumerable permanent benefits.

Isn't it risky to let kids spend their "bonus calories" on any foods they wish—even junk foods?

Absolutely not. The diet plan itself fulfills all of your child's daily requirements. Thus, *whatever* your child decides to spend his calories on, he won't be depriving himself of needed nutrients, nor will he be exceeding the diet's allotted number of calories.

You should certainly encourage your child to spend his bonus calories on healthful foods. However, by allowing your child to spend a modest number of calories on his favorite foods each day, you are teaching him to do what most thin people do: they eat what they like *in moderation.* Bonus calories also provide a small reward to look forward to each day—something that is especially important for children who have trouble keeping a long-term weight-loss goal in focus.

> Measuring serving portions is such a tedious chore. How accurate must the serving sizes be?

It is not necessary to be compulsive about measuring, but you should know that controlling portion size *is* important. Just an extra one hundred calories over a child's daily allowance can mean ten pounds of excess fat at the end of a year.

A good practice is to measure *all* foods at each meal for one week, so that you and your child can become visually accustomed to the various serving sizes. From then on, measure serving portions once every two weeks; unmeasured portions have a way of becoming larger as time goes on.

The following hints can help you to cut down on measuring time:

1. Choose a cup or glass that your child can use at all meals. Measure out four ounces of water in a measuring cup. Pour the water into your child's cup and mark the four-ounce level with masking tape. Repeat this process for eight ounces. Now your child's cup is premeasured.

2. A pork chop which is ¾-inch thick usually weighs about three ounces, once fat and bone are removed.

3. A simple way to measure meat is to read the package label and divide into portions accordingly. For example, a one-pound package of ground meat can easily be divided into eight two-ounce portions, or four four-ounce portions.

4. For diced or canned meats, like Spam, using a liquid measuring cup is quite accurate. Use this method for measuring meat sauces as well.

5. One medium egg equals roughly one ounce of meat.

6. One piece of presliced luncheon meat or American cheese weighs about one ounce.

7. For chicken, one breast or one drumstick and thigh weighs about three ounces.

8. A slice of meat, poultry, or fish about ¼-inch thick and 3 ½ inches by 2 ½ inches equals about one ounce.

9. The USDA publishes a pocket-sized calorie counter, *Calories and Weight,* with an illustrated section on estimating meat portions. Write to the Superintendent of Documents, U.S. Government Printing Office, Washington, D.C., 20402.

> Because my child has been extremely overweight throughout most of his childhood, he has never participated in sports or physical activities. Although he has lost a significant amount of weight, he is still embarrassed about exercising publicly and fears being seen in gym clothes. Is there anything we can do to help him?

I have great empathy for the terror many overweight children feel at the thought of participating in physical education classes. Go to your child's school and enlist the support of his teachers. Explain that your child is on a weight-loss program and under a doctor's care. Request that he be excused from any exercise that is clearly beyond his capability, and from activities that are likely to subject him to ridicule by others. Although you can't do much about the cruelty of your child's peers, you can demand sensitivity of the school staff.

> We both work, and when our son comes home from school, he overeats. What can we do?

It's a great temptation for a child to overeat under these circumstances. He may be tired, or perhaps bored. Often he is not allowed to go out to play, and there is no adult around to scold him if he overindulges. You can help by making nutritious snacks easily available. Reserve a certain area of the refrigerator or cupboard for your child's snack. Have "bonus" foods prearranged and premeasured.

If you can manage it, arrange some enjoyable activity for your child during these after-school hours. He might enjoy a hobby or craft, or some household projects done for pay. If your child is busy and happy, he won't be tempted to break his diet. He will find that eating is one source of pleasure, not the *only* source of pleasure.

At meals, our child is so hungry that he devours his food; he finishes eating in minutes, and looks around for more. Should we give him more to eat?

Your child is not necessarily hungry, he is just accustomed to eating large quantities of food, and consuming it very quickly. Many overweight people get into the habit of eating very rapidly—almost as if they want to gobble the food before they have a chance to feel guilty about it. When people eat in this manner, they often feel unsatisfied even after eating a large meal. This is because their nervous system has not had sufficient time to convey to the brain that their stomach is full and that their nutritional requirements have been met.

You can help prevent this situation by making mealtimes as relaxing and leisurely as possible. Use meals as an occasion for conversation, rather than watching television or eating on the run, as so many families do. Have your child drink water or some other non-caloric beverage at the start of each meal so that he will feel fuller. Encourage him to chew slowly and completely, and to put his fork down between bites. He will be pleasantly surprised at how satisfied he feels and how much more he notices the taste of food when he eats this way.

Do you recommend having my child take diet pills in conjunction with this diet?

I consider diet pills unnecessary and advise against their use. Various consumer groups have urged the government to ban the use of a drug called phenylpropanolamine, which is contained in many nonprescription diet pills, because it has been linked with high blood pressure. It would be nice if there were a pill that could keep us from overeating. However, such a pill does not yet exist.

Our teenage daughter is following the Diet at home, but because she continues to gain weight, we suspect that she's overeating when she goes away from home. What can we do?

This is a common problem with older children (young children seldom have the opportunity to eat secretly because *you* control their diet). Don't accuse your child of cheating: *remember that overeating is not a moral issue.* Nor can you force your child to diet. Simply bring the matter up in a constructive way: "It seems that you're gaining weight. I may be wrong, but you're probably not following the diet when you're away from home. Is there anything we can do to help?"

Depending upon her reply, you might remind your child to complete the ABC exercise when she's tempted to overeat. (See page 50 for information about the ABC technique.) If she resents having to diet, remind her that she won't be on a diet forever. Get her to focus on the long-range benefits of being thin.

Can you offer some general guidelines for preparing foods for my child's diet?

Trim fat from meat and poultry, and use nonstick pans or vegetable sprays rather than butter or oil. Use salt sparingly; while it contains no calories in itself, salt tends to stimulate the appetite, may cause water retention, and has been linked to hypertension. Instead, substitute herbs and spices, or a dash of lemon juice to enhance the flavor of the foods you cook. The recipes in this book use a number of flavorings your family will enjoy in lieu of salt.

My teenager is embarrassed to diet when he is around his friends. Do you have any advice about how he can cope with these social eating situations?

Social eating should not be a problem with the Dachman Diet because your child can eat a wide variety of foods and has bonus calories to spend every day as he wishes. However, there may be times when your child has to refrain from eating while others indulge —times when a diet soda will have to suffice while his friends devour a deep-dish pizza. You might also suggest that willpower and tenacity are nothing to be ashamed of. Assure your child that even though his friends might tease ("Wouldn't you *rather* have a chocolate sundae?"), they will come to respect his courage and strength of character in saying no.

How can I curb my child's craving for sweets?

People seem to be born with a predisposition for sweets. Studies show that even babies prefer sugared water over plain water, and enjoy puddings, strained fruits, and ice cream much more than vegetables or strained meats. This seems a rather strange twist of nature, considering the high caloric content and low nutritional value of sugar.

One solution to this problem is to make use of products such as Equal and Sweet 'N Low. Some recipes and many of the Dachman Diet menu plans incorporate these sweeteners. Most physicians consider these sweeteners to be safe for your child in reasonable amounts. (See page 49 for information on diet sodas and low-calorie sweeteners.) However, if you feel uncomfortable using them, replace them with sugar, and deduct the calories (one teaspoon of sugar equals sixteen calories) from your child's daily bonus allotment.

Your child's preoccupation with sweets is as much habit as craving. Children can learn to enjoy more healthful foods and to become less desirous of candy, cookies, pies, and other types of foods low in nutrition. Fresh fruits have a natural, low-calorie sweet taste and can be sliced, cubed, and frozen for snacks and sugar "attacks."

How can we expect our child to stick to a diet when his friends and relatives tempt him with sweets?

If your child is very young, explain to friends and relatives that your youngster is on a diet and ask them not to give him sweets.

On the other hand, make it clear to an older child that *he* must take responsibility for his own actions. Explain that you cannot and should not intercede every time temptation beckons. Your child should simply inform the friend or relative that he is dieting and that losing weight is very important to him. He will find that most people will respect his efforts and refrain from offering foods.

Although he is losing a pound or two each week, our child is discouraged with his progress, and is beginning to feel that he'll never reach his goal. How can we keep him from giving up?

Tell your child that losing weight is like running in a marathon. A marathon race is more than twenty-six miles long—a great distance to run, but the experienced runner paces himself. When less-experienced runners reach the eleventh mile, they think only of the fifteen miles ahead. They become frustrated and tired, and slow down or drop out. On the other hand, the seasoned marathoner thinks about all the conquered miles, trying to finish each new mile as effectively and efficiently as possible. He takes one mile at a time, and finishes strong. It's very much like the story of the tortoise and the hare: surely and steadily wins the race. With weight loss, *reaching* the goal is much more important than the *time* it takes to reach the goal.

Another way you can help your child cope with the problem of slow progress is to divide the total weight-loss goal into four intermediate goals. Take a picture of your child as he begins the Diet, and again at each intermediate point. As he reaches each goal, celebrate with anything other than food: a movie, something new to wear, tickets to a sporting event. This way, your child's task won't seem so monumental.

Do you recommend low-calorie food substitutes?

Certain low-calorie products can be useful in a diet program. However, you must be vigilant about reading the labels; some so-called "low-calorie" foods contain more calories than you might expect. In addition, many low-calorie foods are no more than chemical look-alikes that may be suspect from a health standpoint.

Should we avoid eating in restaurants with our child while she's on the diet program? We're afraid she will find it difficult to refrain from overeating.

Your child needn't avoid restaurants because she's dieting. Encourage her to plan ahead if you're going out to eat, and perhaps to save her bonus calories (page 75) for this event. As an occasional practice, she might also skip the afternoon snack and add these servings to the restaurant meal.

Choose a restaurant that will prepare food according to your child's needs. If you are unsure whether a restaurant will welcome special requests, simply call ahead.

You and your child can also use the following guide to make menu choices.

Foods to avoid: Avoid sauteed or fried foods, canned fruits, foods with sauces, gravy, or breading. Desserts are best avoided unless you have the bonus calories allotted. If portions are large, request a doggie bag and take the extra food home.

Appetizers: Order vegetable juices, clear soups, fresh vegetables, or dill pickles. Your child may also order shrimp or oysters, but remember to deduct these servings from her meat allowance.

Salads: Vegetable salads or fresh fruit salad (if your child has a fruit allowance for the meal) are good choices. Ask for diet dressing, or for regular dressing to be served on the side.

Vegetables: Order them steamed if possible. If you do order a vegetable with a sauce, have the sauce served on the side.

Breads: Baked, mashed, or boiled potatoes are good choices. Your child may also order a medium-sized dinner roll. (Remember to deduct these servings from her bread allowance.)

Meats: Order meats broiled, roasted, braised, or grilled. Have extra fat trimmed and the skin removed.

Food complements: Your child may request lemon, Tabasco sauce, catsup, or mustard to complement her meal.

Fast foods: If you plan to eat at a fast food restaurant, consult the guide to fast foods included in Appendix 2 (page 217) to calculate serving amounts and calories.

> Watching television seems to trigger our child's urge to snack. Aside from banning TV, do you have any suggestions?

Snacking while watching TV is a ritual in many households, and, like most habits, dies hard. Your child is having difficulty breaking the association between television viewing and absentminded nibbling. It probably doesn't help matters that most commercials which sell sweets and junk foods are aimed directly at kids.

You can help by doing some impromptu consumer education. Explain that advertisers want most of all to sell their product, and not necessarily to promote good health. As you watch commercials, talk about the methods that are used to make food look attractive. Even the youngest child can participate in this kind of discussion. Youngsters often adopt the attitudes of their parents, who are their primary role models, so when you look at a commercial for candy bars or sugar-coated cereal and say, "Yuk! That's junk food—it's really not good for you at all," your preschooler is likely to agree.

> Our child has lost 40 pounds and needs to lose another 65 to reach her ideal weight. However, she is becoming discouraged because her schoolmates don't notice that she's lost weight and still exclude her from activities. How can we assure her that dieting is worth the struggle?

First of all, remind your child that she is losing weight for herself, not for the approval of others; it's her own satisfaction that counts. Eventually, others will notice her weight loss, but social relationships take time and skill to develop, especially if your child has been socially isolated by her weight problem.

I remember going to an ice cream parlor with some of my friends after I had lost a good deal of weight. Even though they ordered hot fudge sundaes and banana splits, I was content to sip on a glass of water because I was feeling so good about my progress.

A group of girls came into the store. I noticed that they were looking my way and giggling. Finally one of them looked at me and said, "What are you doing here, you fat pig?" I was mortified. I thought, "I've tried so hard and lost sixty pounds and I'm still fat; nobody even notices." For a moment I was tempted to order one of those sundaes and give up the whole idea of dieting, but I didn't go off my diet because by now I had become very good at practicing the ABC technique. I realized that if I stayed fat, insensitive people would be taunting me all my life, so I kept losing weight in spite of that girl and ended up reaching my goal. Later, she ended up asking *me* to the senior prom!

6

YOUR NEWLY-THIN CHILD

Staying Thin

ONCE your child has completed the Dachman Diet, he will have changed—he will look better, feel better, and have more energy. By reaching his weight-loss goal, he will have accomplished a feat that should give him greater confidence in his pursuit of other goals.

How can you help your child to *remain* thin? Earlier in this book I promised that your child would not have to diet forever; that in the process of following the Dachman Diet, your youngster would learn many of the strategies he needs to stay thin, perhaps utilizing them without even realizing it. This is exactly as it should be, for, to remain thin, your child must undergo a subtle transformation. *He must come to see himself as a naturally thin person.*

For this reason, I feel a maintenance diet is counterproductive, even destructive; it gives your child the notion that he is still a fat person who temporarily happens to be thin. After all, a maintenance diet is simply a reducing diet with several hundred calories added. If you had to face the prospect of a structured diet for the rest of your life, I'm sure you'd come to the conclusion that losing weight simply wasn't worth the effort. Imagine how grim those endless years of deprivation, stretching far into the future, look to your child!

Do you worry, however, that if your child does not adhere to the structure of a maintenance diet, he will surely lose control? You can stop worrying because when he makes the decision to begin the Dachman Diet, your child will have laid the foundation for a *permanent* weight loss. He will have begun the diet for himself, and he will stay thin for the same reason—any other motive would doom him to failure.

Encouraging Your Child's New Self-Image

How can you be sure that your child will really *feel* like a thin person? Earlier I suggested that you take a picture of your child when she begins the Diet, and, if she had a considerable amount of weight to lose, at intermediate points along the way. Encourage your child to look in the mirror and compare the "old" person to the "new" one.

You can emphasize the change in other ways. Most children who lose a substantial amount of weight begin to take an interest in their appearance for the first time. You should encourage this behavior. Shop with your child for a new wardrobe (this can be a bit expensive, but it's money well spent) or have her try a new hairstyle. Give your child a birthday present that reflects newfound abilities or interests —perhaps roller skates, a new bathing suit, a tennis racket, a bicycle, or lessons in some activity she couldn't manage before.

The diet itself will begin your child's transformation to a thin person. She will become accustomed to eating a balanced diet at regular intervals. She will learn something about foods—what makes up a healthy meal, which foods are high in calories. She'll probably eat a greater variety of foods than before. She will begin to judge eating pleasure not by amount, but by variety. She will also learn, through controlled bonus calories (page 75), that she can eat her favorite foods and still lose weight, and that she can make her own choices.

Checks and Balances

Once your child completes the Diet and sees himself as a thin person, he can learn how his friends remain thin without dieting or depriving themselves of their favorite foods. They do it by monitoring themselves with a system of *checks and balances*.

An older child can often observe this behavior first-hand, as I did. I used to resent the fact that my brothers seemed to be able to eat anything they wanted and still remain thin. After I began to lose weight, I remember watching my brother, Carey, stuff himself full of pizza only an hour or two after eating dinner. When I asked him how he could eat like that and not gain weight, he said, "You're right, I did overeat, but I'll get back on the track in couple of days to make up for it."

This rationale didn't make much sense to me at the time; I just assumed that *my* body handled calories differently from Carey's. As I began to watch more closely, though, I saw the other side of this system of checks and balances. At the local snack shop I ran into my thin neighbor, Mike, who had just come from baseball practice. He had just expended plenty of calories, but after eating a grilled cheese sandwich, he passed up a hot fudge sundae without a moment's hesitation. He explained his behavior by saying, "I know I've worked hard today, but I've had a sandwich and I'm not really hungry. Besides, I'm going to a party tomorrow and I know I'll be eating more than I usually do."

I began to see that there was no insurmountable difference between other children and myself, no miracle that kept them thin. It was ridiculously simple: they "watched" themselves. When they felt they had gained a few pounds, they cut back on their eating for a few days to compensate. One of the benefits of being thin is the ability to gain or lose a few pounds without disastrous results. Because my brother and Mike never let the pounds accumulate, they never faced an overwhelming task when it came to losing them. They kept thin by using an internal system of checks and balances.

Like any new skill, learning to use checks and balances takes some practice. One of the keys to learning thin-person behavior is to establish a *panic point* for your child. Your child's panic point should be a weight perhaps three to five pounds above his ideal weight—a point at which you and he both agree to say, "Oops! Time to do something about this."

Even after your child has completed the Dachman Diet, continue to have him weigh himself twice a week, as he did on the Diet program. In this way, you can monitor his panic point. His weight may fluctuate slightly from week to week, but this is not a matter for concern. However, if he gains enough weight to reach his panic point, your child should immediately cut back on his eating until he returns to his ideal weight.

Your child can lose three to five excess pounds by "watching" himself, just as other thin people do. By paying close attention to what and when he eats, he will soon figure out where the extra calories are coming from. Perhaps he needs to eliminate some high-calorie snacks for the next several days, or to monitor portion sizes at mealtimes. He may also realize that he hasn't been getting as much exercise as he should.

If your youngster finds himself eating at times other than at meals or regular snack times, you should consider the possibility that he may be doing some emotional eating. You can also remind your child to ask himself the ABC questions when he feels tempted to overindulge. (This technique was described in Chapter 5, "Answers To Dieting Questions." See page 50.) If he thinks about the *consequences* of overeating *before* he eats, the chances are good that he won't risk a return to his previous unhappy condition.

Eventually your child may be able to employ checks and balances without weighing himself as often as twice a week. With practice, he will become more sensitive to his body's signals; he'll notice immediately when clothes fit too snugly; he'll learn how to balance eating with exercise. Considering the consequences of overeating *before* the fact will become second nature to him. For the time being, however, it's best to let the scale help your child monitor his weight.

If your child can't seem to "watch" himself back to his proper weight, or is continuing to gain, don't let things snowball. He has worked too hard to become thin to let the pounds creep back now. Have him return to the Dachman Diet until he drops below his panic point again. (Because your child won't need to lose a great deal of weight, you might try a higher level of the diet than he originally followed. Just make sure to calculate his calorie requirements beforehand. Chapter 7, "Getting Started On The Diet," will show you how to do this.) Don't let your child become discouraged; it takes time for new skills to become habits.

7

GETTING STARTED ON
THE DACHMAN DIET

IT is a particularly salient point, in regard to this discussion, that
children have different nutritional and caloric requirements from
adults. While the adult body is simply maintaining itself, the body of a
child is engaged in a constant process of growth and development.
That is why a diet program designed for adults is not appropriate for
children. Additionally, because a child's rate of growth varies a great
deal depending upon his stage of development, a diet for children must
be extremely accurate in determining their caloric needs and flexible
enough to meet those needs.

A restrictive diet which requires a child to begin each morning
with a grapefruit half, or prescribes broccoli every third day, is not
likely to be as successful as a program which offers variety and includes
the types of foods most children enjoy. Youngsters are more likely to
stay with a diet which offers some short-term rewards as they pursue
their long-term weight-loss goals.

About the Dachman Diet

The Dachman Diet has been developed especially for children—to satisfy their tastes as well as their nutritional needs. Your child will be able to *eat* like a child and still lose weight. He will have the freedom to enjoy some of his favorite foods each day. At the same time, however, the scientific design of the Dachman Diet ensures that your child will achieve his ideal weight without compromising healthy growth and development.

Designed to meet the medical standards for caloric and nutritional requirements, the Dachman Diet program is based on seven food groups which are similar to the "basic four" with which you may already be familiar. They are the following:

1. Milk (skim milk, yogurt, dry milk)

2. Meats (fish, red meats, poultry)

3. Breads and Cereals (loaf breads, rolls, crackers, natural cereals, rice)

4. Fruits (any of the fruits and their juices)

5. Vegetables (any of the vegetables)

6. Fats and Oils (margarine, nuts, dressings)

7. Free Foods (low-calorie snack foods)

Structured with three meals and two snacks a day, the Diet is easy to follow. You don't have to count calories; you simply choose *servings* from each of the seven groups.

To provide for the wide range of children's caloric needs, the program offers four levels (A, B, C, and D). Each level follows the same basic pattern, but differs in the number of servings offered at each meal. Each of the four plans includes a 14-day menu featuring foods that most children enjoy: pizza burgers, spaghetti, milkshakes—even a

McDonald's Quarter Pounder. Moreover, your child will have bonus calories to spend each day on foods of his own choosing, from any of the food groups.

The next section of this chapter will show you how to determine which level of the Dachman Diet your child should follow. Because *accuracy is important,* this will require some calculating on your part. You will need to find the number of calories your child needs in order to lose weight in a healthy manner. Once you find this number, choosing the proper level of the Diet is a simple matter.

How Many Calories Does My Child Need?

To determine your child's daily calorie requirement, according to the Dachman Diet, simply divide his *low* ideal weight (see Table 1) by 2.2, and then multiply your answer by the number indicated in Table 2. Subtract 200 from this figure and round off your answer to the nearest decimal point. The formula is really much easier than it sounds, and is well worth this initial effort. The diet starts with this calculation. The formula is broken down and explained to you as follows:

Step 1: Determine your child's ideal weight. (This might be his or her goal.)

Table 1 gives ideal weight ranges for children. These weight ranges are based on your child's height, so it is important that you obtain an accurate measurement. Attach a nonstretchable measuring tape to a wall. Have your child stand barefoot with his back against the tape, heels together. The back of his heels, buttocks, shoulders, and head should be touching the wall. Take his measurement and then locate the proper weight range for your child's height and sex in Table 1. If your child's height exceeds those given in Table 1, simply work with the highest weight range listed. Conversely, if his or her height is less than those given, work with the lowest weight range listed.

Table 1: Chart of Ideal Weights for Children Ages 2 to 18*		
Height In Inches	Weight Range	Weight Range
	For Males	For Females
34-35	25-29	24-28
36-37	27-31	28-32
38-39	30-34	31-35
40-41	33-38	33-38
42-43	35-42	35-43
44-45	40-46	37-45
46-47	42-50	41-50
48-49	46-55	44-54
50-51	50-62	49-62
52-53	55-69	55-70
54-55	62-77	62-82
56-57	67-87	70-93
58-59	75-97	75-99
60-61	81-107	82-107
62-63	89-112	90-118
64-65	98-128	107-135
66-67	109-148	120-135
68-69	122-153	135-145
70-71	130-159	
72-73	160-180	
74-75	170-190	
76-77	190-210	

*From the National Center for Health Statistics Children's Growth Charts, 1984.

To illustrate, let's consider two examples:

For Gina, who is five years old and forty-four inches tall, the ideal weight range is 37 to 45 pounds.

For Mark, age fourteen and sixty-six inches tall, the ideal weight range is 109 to 148 pounds.

Step 2: Use Table 2 to find the calorie equation for your child's sex and age.

Table 2: Recommended Daily Calorie Allowances for Weight Loss*		
Sex	*Age in Years*	*Daily Calorie Equation*
Males and Females	**1-3**	**Low Ideal Weight x 100** over **2.2**
	4-10	**Low Ideal Weight x 85** over **2.2**
Males	**11-14**	**Low Ideal Weight x 60** over **2.2**
	15-18	**Low Ideal Weight x 42** over **2.2**
	19-22	**Low Ideal Weight x 41** over **2.2**
Females	**11-14**	**Low Ideal Weight x 48** over **2.2**
	15-18	**Low Ideal Weight x 38** over **2.2**
	19-22	**Low Ideal Weight x 38** over **2.2**

*From the Committee on Dietary Allowances, Food and Nutrition Board of the National Academy of Sciences, Washington, D.C.

For Gina (female, age 4 to 10), the daily calorie equation would be figured as follows:

$$\frac{\textbf{Low Ideal Weight (37) x 85}}{\textbf{2.2}} = \textbf{1,430 calories}$$

For Mark (male, age 11 to 14), we would use this equation:

$$\frac{\textbf{Low Ideal Weight (109) x 60}}{\textbf{2.2}} = \textbf{2,973 calories}$$

Step 3: Subtract 200 from the figure you arrived at in Step 2. This figure is the number of calories your child needs daily while losing weight.

For Gina: 1,430 — 200 = 1,230 calories per day.

For Mark: 2,973 — 200 = 2,773 calories per day.

Note: If your child is in the teen years, you may be surprised at the large number of calories you have calculated for his daily allowance. You may feel that the allowance is excessive for a weight-loss program—and it would be for an adult—however, adolescents burn large amounts of calories during the period of rapid growth that accompanies puberty. In addition, both young children and teens are usually far more active than adults.

Choosing the Diet: Which Plan Should My Child Follow?

Here's how to determine which level of the Dachman Diet your child should follow. Use column 1 of the following table to find where your child's daily calorie requirement (figured for the Diet) falls by group, and then look under column 2 to find the plan your child should be following.

Number of Daily Calories	Dachman Diet Level
1,100—1,700	Plan A
1,700—2,200	Plan B
2,200—2,800	Plan C
Over 2,800	Plan D

Gina, with a daily requirement of 1,230 calories, would follow Plan A. Mark, who requires 2,773 calories daily, would follow Plan C.

Now that you know how much your child should weigh, how many calories he will require to accomplish this goal, and which diet plan he should follow to achieve that goal, turn to the appropriate diet (These are found in Chapter 8, "The Dachman Diet."). There you will find a 14-day menu plan your child can begin immediately.

How to Follow The Dachman Diet Program with Your Child

If you wish to diet along with your child, follow these steps to determine the number of calories that you need to lose weight safely.

Step 1: Determine your exact height.

Step 2: Determine your ideal body weight. Males should allow 120 pounds for the first 60 inches of height; females should allow 100 pounds. Then add 5 pounds for every inch over 60 inches.

For example, consider Ellen; she is 63 inches tall. Her ideal weight would be figured in this way:

> 100 pounds (for the first 60 inches)
> 63 = 3 inches over 60
> 3 (inches) x 5 pounds (for every inch over 60) = 15 pounds
> 100 (pounds) + 15 (pounds) = Ellen's ideal weight of 115 pounds

Step 3: Multiply your ideal body weight by 10. Then add 200 calories if you have a sedentary lifestyle, or 400 calories if you are moderately active.

Ellen, an active woman, would multiply 115 x 10 (1,150 calories) and add 400 calories for a total of 1,550 calories. Use this final number to determine which level of the Dachman Diet you should follow. Ellen would follow Plan A (1,100-1,700 calories).

8

THE DACHMAN DIET

THIS chapter includes four 14-day menu plans which feature a number of recipes with special appeal for youngsters. (You can find these recipes in Chapter 9, "The Dachman Diet Recipes.") You may wish to begin the Dachman Diet by using one of the 14-day menu plans. After you have acquainted yourself with the patterns for Plans A, B, C, and D, you can easily design a variety of menus yourself, and incorporate many of the Dachman Diet recipes into your own meal plans as well. Appendix 1 (page 209) lists foods by group and indicates the amount that equals one serving. Appendix 1 also lists separately those foods included in the diet plans that are highest in fat content. Foods from the "free" group may be added to any meal as desired.

Bonus Calories

In addition to the number of servings allowed in these daily plans, your child can spend "bonus calories" on foods he enjoys. For instance, if your child's daily calorie requirement is between 1,100 and 1,300 calories, he will have 300 bonus calories to spend. If your child's daily calorie requirement exceeds 1,300 calories, he will have 500 extra calories to spend. *The number of bonus calories available to your child is explained under each diet plan.*

Encourage your child to spend these calories on meats, fruits, or vegetables; however, it is important to let him make his *own* choice. Even if that choice turns out to be a Twinkie (200 calories), potato chips (10 calories apiece), or a chocolate doughnut (135 calories), the structure of the Dachman Diet ensures that your child will not be exceeding his caloric limit or jeopardizing his nutritional requirements.

To help your child keep track of his bonus calories, you should purchase a calorie counter, preferably one which includes brand names and prepared foods for easy reference.

Note: Even if your child follows the prearranged 14-day menu plan, he may still spend his bonus calories!

DIET PLAN A: 1,100-1,700 CALORIES

PLAN A INCLUDES:

6 Milk servings	4 Meat servings	4 Bread servings
3 Fruit serving	1 Vegetable serving	3 Fat servings

BREAKFAST*

1 Milk serving	1 Bread serving	1 Fruit serving

LUNCH

1 Milk serving	2 Meat servings	1 Bread serving
1 Fruit serving		

AFTERNOON SNACK

½ Milk serving	1 Fruit serving

DINNER

½ Milk serving	2 Meat servings	1 Bread serving
1 Vegetable serving	2 Fat servings	

EVENING SNACK

1 Bread serving	1 Fat serving

A vitamin may be given if desired.

* You may wish to include a food from the meat group at breakfast (an egg, for example). If so, simply borrow a meat serving from lunch, dinner, or snacks.

Using Appendix 1 (page 209), you may choose any food from a group in the amount indicated. Either of the following lunches would be appropriate for Plan A.

PATTERN	LUNCH 1	LUNCH 2
1 Milk	Milk (1 cup)	Yogurt (1 cup)
2 Meat	Hot dog (1)	Ham (1 slice)
	Cheese (1 slice)	Cheese (1 slice)
1 Bread	Hot dog bun (1)	Vanilla wafers (5)
1 Fruit	Fruit cocktail	Orange juice
	(½ cup)	(½ cup)
Free foods		Carrot sticks

BONUS CALORIES

If your child's daily calorie requirement is between 1,100 and 1,300 calories, he will have 300 bonus calories to spend. If your child's daily requirement exceeds 1,300 calories, he will have 500 extra calories to spend.

THE DACHMAN DIET RECIPES

Recipes for starred items (*) in the following 14-day menu plan can be found in Chapter 9, "The Dachman Diet Recipes."

DIET PLAN A

DAY 1

BREAKFAST

Orange juice (½ cup)
Graham crackers (2, 2½-inch squares) **in skim milk** (1 cup)

LUNCH

Sandwich: Bologna (2 slices); Lettuce, tomato, mustard (as desired); Whole wheat bread (1 slice)
Green grapes (24, small)
Hot Chocolate Skim Milk* (1 cup)

AFTERNOON SNACK

Vanilla Yogurt* (½ cup) **over sliced banana** (½, small)

DINNER

Spaghetti: Peppy Spaghetti Sauce* (1 serving) Noodles (4 ounces)
Salad (as desired)
Low-Cal Thousand Island Dressing* (2 servings)
Skim milk (½ cup)

EVENING SNACK

Rice Krispie Square* (1)
Diet Kool-Aid of choice (as desired)
Cream Cheese Frosting* (1 serving)

DIET PLAN A

DAY 2

BREAKFAST

Cinnamon applesauce (½ cup sauce, dash cinnamon)
Golden Pancake* (1)
Special Syrup* (as desired)
Skim milk (1 cup)

LUNCH

Sandwich: Sliced banana (½, small), Diet jelly (2 tablespoons), Whole wheat bread (1 slice)
String cheese (2 ounces)
Skim milk (1 cup)

AFTERNOON SNACK

Raisins (2 tablespoons)
Skim milk (1 cup)

DINNER

Dog 'n' Beans (¾ hot dog, 2 ounces pork 'n' beans)
Wax beans (½ cup) **with diet margarine** (2 teaspoons)
Green pepper slices (as desired)
Skim milk (½ cup)
Saltine crackers (3)

EVENING SNACK

Jelly Drop* (1)
Diet soda of choice (as desired)

DIET PLAN A

DAY 3

BREAKFAST

Grape juice (¼ cup)
Cheerios (¾ cup) **with low-calorie sweetener** (as desired)
Skim milk (1 cup)

LUNCH

Creamy soup (1 serving)
Oyster crackers (10)
Summer sausage roll (2 slices sausage, rolled with lettuce and mustard)
Apple boats (1 apple, quartered)
Hot Chocolate Skim Milk* (1 cup)

AFTERNOON SNACK

Strawberry Ice* (1 serving)

DINNER

Roast beef (2 ounces)
Corn on the cob (1, about 4 inches long)
Diet margarine (4 teaspoons)
Green pepper and celery with All-Purpose French Dressing* (as desired)
Tomato juice (½ cup)
Skim milk (½ cup)

EVENING SNACK

Potato chips (10)

DIET PLAN A

DAY 4

BREAKFAST

English muffin (½ muffin)
Orange-Raisin Spread* (1 serving)
Skim milk (1 cup)

LUNCH

Finger sandwiches: Sausage (2 ounces), Cocktail rye bread (3 slices), Cherry tomatoes (2, sliced)
Tangerine slices (1 tangerine)
Hot Chocolate Skim Milk* (1 cup)

AFTERNOON SNACK

Orange Slush* (2 servings)
Fruit roll-up (½)

DINNER

Cheesy Macaroni* (1 serving)
Green beans (½ cup)
Diet margarine (2 teaspoons)
Skim milk (½ cup)

EVENING SNACK

Salty Corn Chips* (1 serving)
Onion Dip* (1 serving)
Diet Kool-Aid of choice (as desired)

DIET PLAN A

DAY 5

BREAKFAST

Sliced banana (½, small) **in skim milk** (1 cup) **topped with cinnamon and low-calorie sweetener**
Toast dunkers (1 slice toast, quartered)

LUNCH

Spaghettios (3 ounces) **with hot dog slices** (2 ounces)
Lime-Applesauce Gelatin* (1 serving)
Skim milk (1 cup)

AFTERNOON SNACK

Hot Chocolate Skim Milk* (½ cup)
Banana (½, small)

DINNER

Hamburger Stew* (1 serving)
Baked potato (1, small)
Sour half-and-half (4 tablespoons), **or diet margarine** (2 tablespoons)
Vanilla Yogurt* (½ cup)

EVENING SNACK

Oven Fries* (1 serving)
Diet Kool-Aid of choice (as desired)

DIET PLAN A

DAY 6

BREAKFAST

Fruity Milk* (1 serving)
Graham crackers (2, 2½-inch squares)

LUNCH

Sandwich: Hot dog (1, 2-ounce) wrapped in crescent roll; Pickles, catsup, mustard (as desired)
Chocolate skim milk (1 cup)

AFTERNOON SNACK

Diet Orange Soda Fizzy* (½ serving)
Cinnamon applesauce (½ cup)

DINNER

Baked chicken (2 ounces, or 1 drumstick)
Mashed Squash* (1 serving)
Diet margarine (2 teaspoons)
Coleslaw* (½ cup)
Skim milk (½ cup)

EVENING SNACK

Maple Custard* (1 serving)
Cream Cheese Frosting* (1 serving)

DIET PLAN A

DAY 7

BREAKFAST

Orange slices (½ orange)
Biscuit Kalacky* (1)
Skim milk (1 cup)

LUNCH

Sandwich: Egg Salad* (1 serving), Whole wheat bread (1 slice)
Cherry Opaque Gelatin* (1 serving)
Grape Natural Fruit Soda* (1 serving)
Cheesy Celery* (1 serving)

AFTERNOON SNACK

Aloha Fruit Salad* (½ cup)
Skim milk (½ cup)

DINNER

Beef Stroganoff* (1 serving)
Green beans (½ cup)
Diet margarine (2 teaspoons)
Sliced bell pepper (1, small) **with All-Purpose French Dressing*** (as desired)
Skim milk (½ cup)

EVENING SNACK

Toasted English muffin (½ muffin) **with diet margarine** (2 teaspoons) **and cinnamon**

DIET PLAN A

DAY 8

BREAKFAST

Banana (½, small)
Applesauce Muffin* (1)
Diet jelly (2 teaspoons)
Skim milk (1 cup)

LUNCH

Scrambled eggs (2 eggs)
Plums (2, small)
Vanilla wafers (5)
Skim milk (1 cup)

AFTERNOON SNACK

Aloha Fruit Salad* (1 serving)
Skim milk (½ cup)

DINNER

Turkey breast roll (2 ounces)
Stuffing* (½ serving)
Chicken and Parsley Rice* (¼ cup)
Almond Green Beans* (¼ cup)
Diet margarine (2 teaspoons)

EVENING SNACK

Popcorn-Pretzel Mix* (1 serving)
Lemonade* (as desired)

DIET PLAN A

DAY 9

BREAKFAST

Crunchy Apple-Raisin Oatmeal* (1 serving)
Skim milk (1 cup)

LUNCH

Cherry Opaque Gelatin* (1 serving)
Hors d'oeuvres* with Rye Crisp crackers (1 serving) **and parsley garnish**
(to taste)
Grape juice (¼ cup)

AFTERNOON SNACK

Raisins (1 tablespoon)
Strawberry Yogurt* (½ serving)

DINNER

Sloppy Joes* (1 serving meat, ½ bun)
Sauteed Mushrooms or Onions* (1 serving)
Green pepper and tomato salad (as desired) **with Low-Cal Thousand
Island Dressing*** (1 serving)
Skim milk (½ cup)

EVENING SNACK

Coconut-Rice Pudding* (1 serving)
Diet Kool-Aid of choice (as desired)

DIET PLAN A

DAY 10

BREAKFAST

Strawberry Yogurt* (1 serving)
Graham crackers (2, 2½-inch squares)

LUNCH

Sandwich: Pizza Burger* (½ serving) on English Muffin
Chilled apricots (4 halves)
Chocolate Skim Milk* (½ cup)

AFTERNOON SNACK

Watermelon balls (1 cup)
Skim milk (½ cup)
Popcorn with butter buds (as desired)

DINNER

Hamburger Stew* (1 serving)
Fried Rice* (1 serving)
Diet margarine (2 teaspoons)
Lime-Carrot Mold* with All-Purpose French Dressing* (as desired)
(Variation on Fruit Salad Mold*)
Skim milk (½ cup)

EVENING SNACK

Chocolate-Coconut Drops* (1 serving)
Diet soda of choice (as desired)

DIET PLAN A

DAY 11

BREAKFAST

Pineapple chunks (½ cup) **on Cinnamon French Toast*** (1 serving)
Special Syrup* (as desired)
Skim milk (1 cup)

LUNCH

Sandwich: Grilled Cheese Plus* (1 slice cheese)
Strawberries (¾ cup)
Diet Root Beer Fizzy* (1 serving)

AFTERNOON SNACK

Fruity Milk* (½ serving)
Popcorn with butter buds (as desired)
Apple (½, sliced)

DINNER

Cube steak (2 ½ ounces)
Gravy noodles (½ cup noodles, ¼ cup gravy)
Zucchini Fingers* (½ cup)
Orange Opaque Gelatin* (1 serving)
Lemonade* (as desired)

EVENING SNACK

Cheesy Jelly Toast* (1 serving)
Lemonade* (as desired)

DIET PLAN A

DAY 12

BREAKFAST
Sliced banana (½, small) **in cornflakes** (¾ cup)
Skim milk (1 cup)

LUNCH
Ham 'n' Cheese Roll-Up* (1 serving)
Pretzel sticks (20, small)
Raisins (2 tablespoons)
Skim milk (1 cup)

AFTERNOON SNACK
Orange Slush* (2 servings)
Pear (½, small)

DINNER
Baked Fish* (2 ounces)
Cottage fries (8 slices)
Diet margarine (2 teaspoons)
Boiled cabbage (½ cup) **in Paprika White Sauce*** (1 serving)
Cherry Opague Gelatin* (1 serving)
Diet Orange Soda Fizzy* (1 serving)

EVENING SNACK
Salty Corn Chips* (1 serving)
Onion Dip* (1 serving)

DIET PLAN A

DAY 13

BREAKFAST

Fruit cocktail (½ cup)
Cinnamon Toast* (1 slice)
Skim milk (1 cup)

LUNCH

Cheeseburger Patty (½ slice cheese, 1½ ounces meat)
Oven Fries* (1 serving)
Raspberry Opaque Gelatin* (1 serving)
Orange juice (½ cup)

AFTERNOON SNACK

Pretty Pastel Cookies* (2 servings)
Banana (½, small)

DINNER

Baked Cornflake Chicken* (1 drumstick)
Chicken and Parsley Rice* (½ cup)
Wax beans (½ cup)
Diet margarine (2 teaspoons)
Tomato slices with All-Purpose French Dressing* (as desired)
Skim milk (½ cup)

EVENING SNACK

Applesauce Muffin* (1)
Diet Kool-Aid of choice (as desired)

DIET PLAN A

DAY 14

BREAKFAST

Orange slices (1 orange)
Lemony Vanilla Pudding* (1 serving)
Grape juice (¼ cup)

LUNCH

Salad: Cottage cheese (½ cup) and Aloha Fruit Salad* (1 serving)
Vanilla wafers (5)
Soda Fizzy* (1 serving)

AFTERNOON SNACK

Fruit Salad Mold* (1 serving)
Skim milk (½ cup)

DINNER

Chicken and Broccoli Casserole* (1 serving)
Lettuce salad (as desired) **with Low-Cal Thousand Island Dressing*** (2 servings)
Hot roll (1) **with diet margarine** (2 teaspoons)
Diet Kool-Aid of choice (as desired)

EVENING SNACK

Graham crackers (2, 2½-inch squares) **with Cream Cheese Frosting*** (1 serving)

DIET PLAN B: 1,700-2,200 CALORIES

PLAN B INCLUDES:

3 Milk servings	7 Meat servings	6 Bread servings
3 Fruit servings	2 Vegetable servings	3 Fat servings

BREAKFAST*

1 Milk serving	2 Bread servings	1 Fruit serving
1 Fat serving		

LUNCH

1 Milk serving	3 Meat servings	2 Bread servings
1 Fruit serving		

AFTERNOON SNACK

1 Fruit serving

DINNER

1 Milk serving	3 Meat servings	1 Bread serving
2 Vegetable servings	1 Fat serving	

EVENING SNACK

1 Meat serving	1 Bread serving	1 Fat serving

A vitamin can be given if desired.

* You may wish to include a food from the meat group at breakfast (an egg, for example). If so, simply borrow a meat serving from lunch, dinner, or snacks.

Using Appendix 1 (page 209), you may choose any food from a group in the amount indicated. Either of the following lunches would be appropriate for Plan B.

PATTERN	LUNCH 1	LUNCH 2
1 Milk	Milk (1 cup)	Yogurt (1 cup)
3 Meat	Grilled cheese w/ham (2 slices cheese)	Roast beef (2 slices)
2 Bread	Bread (2 slices)	Bread (2 slices)
1 Fruit	Apple (1)	Orange (1)
Free foods	Carrot sticks	Diet soda

BONUS CALORIES

If your child's daily calorie requirement is between 1,700 and 1,900 calories, he will have 300 bonus calories to spend. If your child's daily requirement exceeds 1,900 calories, he will have 500 extra calories to spend.

THE DACHMAN DIET RECIPES

Recipes for starred items (*) in the following 14-day menu plan can be found in Chapter 9, "The Dachman Diet Recipes."

DIET PLAN B

DAY 1

BREAKFAST

Orange juice (½ cup)
Golden Pancakes* (2)
Special Syrup* (as desired)
Skim milk (1 cup)

LUNCH

Sandwich: Ham (2 slices) and cheese (1 slice); Whole wheat bread (2 slices); Lettuce, tomato, mustard (as desired)
Pear halves (2)
Chocolate Skim Milk* (1 cup)

AFTERNOON SNACK

Popsicle (1)

DINNER

Spaghetti (4 ounces) **and Peppy Spaghetti Sauce*** (1 serving)
Green beans (½ cup)
Skim milk (1 cup)

EVENING SNACK

Salty Corn Chips* (1 serving)
Johnny C's Spicy Sauce* (as desired)
Orange juice (½ cup)

DIET PLAN B

DAY 2

BREAKFAST

Banana (½, small)
Raisin bran (½ cup)
Whole wheat toast (1 slice)
Diet jelly (1 teaspoon)
Diet margarine (2 teaspoons)
Skim milk (1 cup)

LUNCH

Polish sausage (3 ounces) **on hot dog bun**
Dill pickles (as desired)
Strawberry Fruity Milk* (1 serving)

AFTERNOON SNACK

Natural Fruit Soda* (1 serving)
Popcorn with butter buds (as desired)

DINNER

Barbecued Ribs Or Chicken* (1 serving)
Creamy Tomato Soup* (1 cup)
Saltine crackers (3)
Broccoli (½ cup)
Skim milk (½ cup)
Diet Kool-Aid of choice (as desired)

EVENING SNACK

Sandwich: bologna (1 slice), Whole wheat bread (1 slice), Lettuce and mustard (as desired)
Sauteed Mushrooms Or Onions* (1 serving)

DIET PLAN B

DAY 3

BREAKFAST

Poached egg (1, medium-sized)
English muffin (1)
Diet margarine (2 teaspoons)
Orange-Raisin Spread* (2 tablespoons)
Skim milk (1 cup)

LUNCH

Sandwich: Peanut butter (1 tablespoon), Diet jelly (2 teaspoons), Whole wheat bread (1 slice)
Cheesy Celery* (2 servings)
Lorna Doone cookies (3)
Skim milk (1 cup)

AFTERNOON SNACK

Pear-Half Gelatin* (1 serving. See recipe for Fruit Salad Mold)
Lemonade* (as desired)

DINNER

Pork Chow Mein* (1 serving)
Rice (¼ cup)
Chow mein noodles (¼ cup)
Skim milk (1 cup)

EVENING SNACK

Bagel (½)
Salami (1 slice)
Low-calorie cream cheese (2 tablespoons)
Orange juice (½ cup)

DIET PLAN B

DAY 4

BREAKFAST

Cinnamon French Toast* (1 serving)
Diet margarine (2 teaspoons)
Special Syrup* (as desired)
Applesauce (¼ cup)
Vanilla Yogurt* (1 serving)

LUNCH

Soft Shell Tacos* (1 serving)
Banana Fruity Milk* (1 serving)
Lime-Applesauce Gelatin* (as desired)

AFTERNOON SNACK

Orange Natural Fruit Soda* (1 serving)

DINNER

Baked fish fillet (2½ ounces)
Corn on the cob (1, about 4 inches long)
Spinach (1 cup) **in Paprika White Sauce*** (½ cup)
Hot Chocolate Skim Milk* (½ cup)

EVENING SNACK

Potato Skins* (1 serving) **with Lite Line cheese** (1½ slices, melted over skins)

DIET PLAN B

DAY 5

BREAKFAST

Orange slices (½ orange)
Raisin toast (2 slices)
Diet margarine (2 teaspoons)
Orange-Pineapple Milkshake* (1 serving)

LUNCH

Hot sandwich: Cheeseburger (1 ounce cheese, 2 ounces beef), Bun (1)
Pear-Half Gelatin* (1 serving. See recipe for Fruit Salad Mold)
Skim milk (1 cup)

AFTERNOON SNACK

Apple slices (1 apple)

DINNER

Broiled steak (3 ounces)
Baked potato (1, small) **with sour cream** (2 tablespoons), **or diet margarine** (2 teaspoons)
Lemon broccoli (1 cup, with lemon as desired)
Skim milk (1 cup)

EVENING SNACK

Deviled Egg* (1)
Diet soda of choice (as desired)
Saltine crackers (6)

DIET PLAN B

DAY 6

BREAKFAST

Pink grapefruit (½)
Graham crackers (4, 2½-inch squares) **in skim milk** (1 cup)

LUNCH

Hot sandwich: Pizza Burger* (1 serving) on hamburger bun
Grapes (24, small)
Pretzel sticks (20, small)
Diet Lemon-Lime Soda Fizzy* (1 serving)

AFTERNOON SNACK

Fruit roll-up (1)

DINNER

Ham Hash* (1½ servings)
Spicy Carrots* (1 serving)
Tomato juice (½ cup)
Diet Kool-Aid of choice (as desired)

EVENING SNACK

Sausage patty (1)
English muffin (½)
Diet soda of choice (as desired)
Diet margarine (2 teaspoons)

DIET PLAN B

DAY 7

BREAKFAST

Grapes (12, large)
Chocolate Cream of Wheat (½ cup) **with low-calorie sweetener**
(as desired)
English muffin (½)
Diet margarine (2 teaspoons)
Skim milk (1 cup)

LUNCH

Sandwich: Salami (3 slices); Poppy seed bun (1); Lettuce, tomato, mustard, dill pickle
(as desired)
Cantaloupe (¼ small)
Skim milk (1 cup)

AFTERNOON SNACK

Banana (½ small)

DINNER

Chop Suey* (1 serving)
Green beans (½ cup)
Raw mushrooms (or lettuce) **with All-Purpose French Dressing*** (as desired)
Diet Strawberry Soda Fizzy* (½ serving)

EVENING SNACK

Cottage Cheese Cake* (1 serving) **with Tip Top Strawberry Sauce*** (2 servings)
Vanilla wafers (5)

DIET PLAN B

DAY 8

BREAKFAST

Biscuits Kalacky* (2)
Diet margarine (2 teaspoons)
Skim milk (1 cup)

LUNCH

Cheesy dog sandwich: Hot dog (2 ounces), Lite Line cheese (1 slice), Bun (1)
Orange and pineapple fruit salad (½ cup) **with Tip Top**
Strawberry Sauce* (1 serving)
Skim milk (1 cup)

AFTERNOON SNACK

Deviled Egg* (1)
Wheat Thins (6)
Diet Kool-Aid of choice (as desired)

DINNER

Ginger Pork Chops* (3 ounces)
Oriental vegetables (1 cup)
Mashed Squash* (1 serving)
Stewed tomato salad (1 cup) **with All-Purpose French Dressing***
(as desired)
Hot Chocolate Skim Milk* (1 cup)

EVENING SNACK

Peach Gelatin* (1 serving. See recipe for Fruit Salad Mold)
Diet Kool-Aid of choice (as desired)

DIET PLAN B

DAY 9

BREAKFAST

Poached egg (1, medium-sized) **on English muffin** (½, toasted)
Low-sugar cereal (½ cup) **with strawberries** (¾ cup) **and low-calorie sweetener** (as desired)
Skim milk (1 cup)

LUNCH

Hot sandwich: Tuna (2 ounces, water-packed), Pita bread (1 slice), Raw sliced onions (as desired), All-Purpose French Dressing* (as desired)
Vanilla Yogurt* (1 serving)
Orange juice (½ cup)

AFTERNOON SNACK

Tangerine (1)
Vanilla Coke* (as desired)

DINNER

Lasagna* (1 serving)
Wax beans (½ cup)
Green pepper and lettuce salad with All-Purpose French Dressing* (as desired)
Chocolate skim milk* (1 cup)

EVENING SNACK

Oven Fries* (1 serving) **covered with melted cheese** (1 slice)
Diet Kool-Aid of choice (as desired)

DIET PLAN B

DAY 10

BREAKFAST

Bagel (1, toasted)
Diet margarine (2 teaspoons)
Orange-Raisin Spread* (1 serving)
Skim milk (1 cup)

LUNCH

Sandwich: Roast beef (2 ounces); Rye bread (2 slices); Lettuce, tomato, horseradish, mustard (as desired)
Dill pickles (as desired)
Cheesy Pear Salad* (1 serving)
Skim milk (1 cup)

AFTERNOON SNACK

Orange Natural Fruit Soda* (1 serving)
Popcorn with butter buds (as desired)

DINNER

Olé Toro Chili* (1 serving) **in green pepper shell** (1 large pepper. See recipe for Stuffed Green Peppers*)
Lettuce salad (as desired) **with Low-Cal Thousand Island Dressing*** (2 tablespoons)
Strawberry Opaque Gelatin* (1 serving)
Lemonade* (as desired)

EVENING SNACK

Sandwich: Egg (1, medium-sized) fried in diet margarine (2 teaspoons), Whole wheat bread (1 slice), Catsup (1 tablespoon)

DIET PLAN B

DAY 11

BREAKFAST

Orange juice (½ cup)
Lemony Vanilla Pudding* (1 serving)
Bagel (1, toasted)
Diet margarine (2 teaspoons)

LUNCH

Creamy Tomato Soup* (1 serving)
Oyster crackers (10)
Celery stuffed with liver sausage (3 ounces meat)
Vanilla Yogurt* (1 serving)
Apple (1)
Iced tea with lemon (as desired)

AFTERNOON SNACK

Fruit roll-up (1)
Diet soda of choice (as desired)

DINNER

Roast beef (3 ounces)
Mashed potato (½ cup) **with gravy** (1 ounce)
Broccoli (1 cup)
Skim milk (1 cup)

EVENING SNACK

Sandwich: Fancy Taco: Sliced roast beef (1 ounce); Soft shell tortilla (1); Lettuce, tomato, onion (as desired); Sour cream (2 tablespoons); Johnny C's Spicy Sauce***** (as desired)

DIET PLAN B

DAY 12

BREAKFAST

Orange juice (½ cup)
Shredded Wheat (½ cup) **with low-calorie sweetener** (as desired)
Raisin toast (1 slice)
Diet margarine (2 teaspoons)
Skim milk (1 cup)

LUNCH

Sandwich: Grilled Cheese Plus* (1 serving) with ham (1 slice)
Strawberry Yogurt* (1 serving)
Pear-Strawberry Gelatin* (1 serving. See recipe for Fruit Salad Mold*)
Vanilla Cola* (as desired)

AFTERNOON SNACK

Pear (1)
Diet soda of choice (as desired)

DINNER

Baked ham (3 ounces)
Chicken and Parsley Rice* (½ cup)
Ratatouille Royal* (1 serving)
Skim milk (1 cup)

EVENING SNACK

Sandwich: Cheese (1 slice), Tomato (as desired), Whole wheat bread (1 slice),
Diet mayonnaise (1 teaspoon)

DIET PLAN B

DAY 13

BREAKFAST

Chilled pears (2 halves)
Applesauce Muffins* (2)
Diet margarine (2 teaspoons)
Skim milk (1 cup)

LUNCH

Cottage Cheese and Tomato Salad* (2 servings)
Rye Crisp crackers (4)
Fruit Salad Mold* with Tip Top Strawberry Sauce* (1 serving each)
Eggnog* (1 serving)

AFTERNOON SNACK

Aloha Fruit Salad* (1 serving)

DINNER

Meat Loaf* (1 serving)
Wax beans (½ cup) **in Paprika White Sauce*** (1 serving)
Tomato slices (as desired) **with Low-Cal Thousand Island Dressing*** (2 servings)
Skim milk (½ cup)

EVENING SNACK

Ham slice (1 ounce)
Pudding popsicle (1)
Orange Natural Fruit Soda* (1 serving)

DIET PLAN B

DAY 14

BREAKFAST

Sandwich: Banana strips (½ small banana), Whole wheat toast (2 slices), Diet jelly (2 teaspoons), Diet margarine (2 teaspoons)
Skim milk (1 cup)

LUNCH

Hot sandwich: Soft Shell Taco* (1 serving)
Fruit cocktail (½ cup)
Skim milk (1 cup)

AFTERNOON SNACK

Fruit roll-up (1)
Popcorn with butter buds (as desired)

DINNER

Pork roast (3 ounces)
Baked sweet potato (½ small)
Cauliflower (1 cup)
Diet margarine (2 teaspoons)
Lime sugar free gelatin (as desired, see recipe for Fruit Salad Mold.*)
Hot chocolate* (1 serving. See recipe for Fruity Milk*)

EVENING SNACK

Saltine crackers (6)
Lite Line cheese (1½ slices)
Popsicle (1)

DIET PLAN C: 1 2,200-2,800 CALORIES

PLAN C INCLUDES:

3 Milk servings	8 Meat servings	13 Bread servings
5 Fruit servings	2 Vegetable servings	4 Fat servings

BREAKFAST*

1 Milk serving	3 Bread servings	3 Fruit servings
1 Fat serving		

LUNCH

1 Milk serving	3 Meat servings	3 Bread servings
1 Fruit serving	1 Fat serving	

AFTERNOON SNACK

1 Fruit serving

DINNER

1 Milk serving	3 Meat servings	1 Bread serving
2 Vegetable servings	1 Fat serving	

EVENING SNACK

1 Meat serving	1 Bread serving	1 Fat serving

A vitamin can be given if desired.

*You may wish to include a food from the meat group at breakfast (an egg, for example). If so, simply borrow a meat serving from lunch, dinner, or snacks.

Using Appendix 1 (page 209), you may choose any food from a group in the amount indicated. Either of the following lunches would be appropriate for Plan C.

PATTERN	LUNCH 1	LUNCH 2
1 Milk	Milk (1 cup)	Yogurt (1 cup)
3 Meat	Brick cheese (1 slice)	Hot dog (1)
	Salami (2 slices)	Cheese (2 slices)
3 Bread	Bread (2 slices)	Hot dog bun (1)
1 Fruit	Ice cream (½ cup)	Vanilla wafers (5)
1 Fat	Peach (1, sliced)	Apple (1)
	Used in ice cream	Used with hot dog
Free foods		Carrot sticks

BONUS CALORIE

If your child's daily calorie requirement is between 2,300 and 2,500 calories, he will have 300 bonus calories to spend. If your child's daily requirement exceeds 2,500 calories, he will have 500 extra calories to spend.

THE DACHMAN DIET RECIPES

Recipes for the starred items (*) in the following 14-day menu plan can be found in Chapter 9, "The Dachman Diet Recipes."

DIET PLAN C

DAY 1

BREAKFAST

Orange juice (1 cup)
Bran Chex (½ cup) **with sliced banana** (½ small)
Raisin toast (2 slices)
Diet jelly (2 teaspoons)
Skim milk (1 cup)

LUNCH

Hot sandwich: Cheeseburger (1 ounce cheese, 2 ounces meat), Bun (1)
Sauteed Mushrooms or Onions* (1 serving)
Salty Corn Chips* (1 serving)
Apple (1)
Skim milk (1 cup)

AFTERNOON SNACK

Saucy Apple Cake* (2 servings)
Iced tea with lemon (as desired)

DINNER

Spaghetti (8 ounces) **with Peppy Spaghetti Sauce*** (2 servings)
Lettuce salad with All-Purpose French Dressing* (as desired)
Italian Loaf Bread* (1 slice)
Diet Root Beer Fizzy* (1 serving. See Soda Fizzy*)

EVENING SNACK

Sandwich: Lite Line cheese (1½ slices); Whole wheat bread (2 slices); Tomato, horseradish, mustard (as desired)
Dill pickles (as desired)
Diet soda of choice (as desired)

DIET PLAN C

DAY 2

BREAKFAST

Applesauce Muffins* (3 servings)
Diet jelly (2 teaspoons)
Diet margarine (2 teaspoons)
Orange-Raisin Spread* (2 servings)
Strawberry Yogurt* (1 serving)

LUNCH

Sandwich: Cheese (1 slice); Salami (2 ounces); Whole wheat bread (2 slices); Diet mayonnaise (1 teaspoon); Lettuce, mustard (as desired)
Rice Krispie Square* (1)
Apple (1)
Skim milk (1 cup)

AFTERNOON SNACK

Cottage Cheese Cake* (1 serving) **with Tip Top Strawberry Sauce*** (1 serving)
Vanilla wafers (3)

DINNER

Baked ham (4 ounces)
Baked sweet potato (1, medium-sized)
Brussels sprouts (1 cup)
Diet margarine (2 teaspoons)
Lemon sugar-free gelatin (as desired)
Skim milk (1 cup)

EVENING SNACK

Bagel (1)
Cream cheese (1 tablespoon)
Orange juice (½ cup)

DIET PLAN C

DAY 3

BREAKFAST

Orange juice (1 cup)
Blueberries (½ cup)
Golden Pancakes* (3)
Special Syrup* (as desired)
Skim milk (1 cup)

LUNCH

Hot sandwich: Reuben* (1 serving)
Grapes (24, small)
Vanilla wafers (5)
Skim milk (1 cup)

AFTERNOON SNACK

Campbell's Mac 'n' Beef in Tomato Sauce (7½-ounce serving)
Vanilla Coke* (as desired)

DINNER

Pork and Beans* (1 serving)
Broccoli (1 cup)
Dinner rolls (2)
Cherry sugar-free gelatin (as desired)
Skim milk (1 cup)

EVENING SNACK

Saltine crackers (6)
Orange-Raisin Spread* (1 serving)
Diet soda of choice (as desired)

DIET PLAN C

DAY 4

BREAKFAST

Grape juice (¾ cup)
Sandwich: Sausage patty (1 ounce), English muffin (1)
Cheerios (¾ cup) **with low-calorie sweetener** (as desired)
Skim milk (1 cup)

LUNCH

Cheesy Macaroni* (1 serving)
Fruit cocktail (½ cup)
Pumpkin Pie* (2 slices)
Skim milk (½ cup)

AFTERNOON SNACK

Sandwich: Open-faced grilled cheese (1½ ounces Lite Line cheese); Whole wheat bread (2 slices); Mustard, catsup, onion (as desired)
Diet soda of choice

DINNER

Oven Swiss Steak* (4 ounces)
Oniony Noodles* (4 ounces)
Spinach (1 cup) **with lemon** (as desired)
Pillsbury buttermilk biscuits (2)
Diet jelly (2 teaspoons)
Diet margarine (2 teaspoons)
Skim milk (1 cup)

EVENING SNACK

Hostess Ding Dong (1)
Popcorn with butter buds (as desired)
Iced tea with lemon (as desired)

DIET PLAN C

DAY 5

BREAKFAST

Fried Apple Slices* (1 serving)
Oatmeal (½ cup) **with low-calorie sweetener** (as desired)
Egg bagel (1)
Orange-Raisin Spread* (2 servings)
Skim milk (1 cup)

LUNCH

McDonald's Quarter Pounder (1)
Tangerine (1)
Lorna Doone cookies (3)
Skim milk (1 cup)

AFTERNOON SNACK

Chicken noodle soup (1 cup)
Oyster crackers (20)
Diet Kool-Aid of choice (as desired)

DINNER

Cornflake Chicken* (1 serving)
Corn on the cob (8 inches long)
Snappy Ham Beans (2 servings. See recipe for Snappy Bacon Beans*)
Tomato and green pepper salad with All-Purpose French Dressing* (as desired)
Skim milk (1 cup)

EVENING SNACK

Float: Diet soda of choice (as desired), Vanilla ice cream (1/2 cup)
Vanilla wafers (3)

DIET PLAN C

DAY 6

BREAKFAST

Orange juice (1 cup)
Crunchy Apple-Raisin Oatmeal* (1 serving) **with low-calorie sweetener**
English muffin (1)
Diet margarine (2 teaspoons)
Skim milk (1 cup)

LUNCH

Sandwich: Italian beef (3 ounces), Italian bread (2 slices, about 4 inches long), Fat-free beef broth (as desired)
Carrot sticks (as desired)
Strawberry Shortcake* (1 serving)
Skim milk (1 cup)

AFTERNOON SNACK

Sandwich: Egg (1, over easy, use vegetable pan spray), Barbecue sauce (2 teaspoons), Whole wheat bread (2 slices)
Diet soda of choice (as desired)

DINNER

Ham 'n' Eggs* (2 servings)
Toast (2 slices) **with diet jelly** (2 teaspoons)
Ratatouille Royal* (1 serving)
Freezer Fudge Bar* (1)
Skim milk (1 cup)

EVENING SNACK

Saltine crackers (6)
Creamy Tomato Soup* (2 servings)
Apple juice (3 ounces)

DIET PLAN C

DAY 7

BREAKFAST

Breakfast Yogurt: Plain yogurt (1 cup),Sunflower seeds (1 tablespoon), Dates (3, chopped), Raisins (3 tablespoons), Vanilla and low-calorie sweetener (as desired)
Rice Krispie Squares* (3)
Lemonade* (as desired)

LUNCH

Individual Pizzas* (3 servings)
Grapes (24, small)
Diet Orange Fizzy* (1 serving)

AFTERNOON SNACK

Franco-American Mac 'n' Beef (7½ ounces)
Diet soda of choice (as desired)

DINNER

Tuna Loaf* (1 serving)
Corn Casserole* (1 serving)
Ice milk of choice (3/4 cup) **with Tip Top Strawberry Sauce***
(1 serving)
Vanilla wafers (2)

EVENING SNACK

Toast (2 slices)
Diet jelly (2 teaspoons)
Diet margarine (4 teaspoons)
Grapefruit (½)
Diet Kool-Aid of choice (as desired)

DIET PLAN C

DAY 8

BREAKFAST

Grape juice (½ cup)
Egg (1, medium-sized) **and Bacon** (2 slices)
Whole wheat toast (3 slices) **with diet jelly** (3 tablespoons)
Grapefruit (½)
Skim milk (1 cup)

LUNCH

Sandwich: Francheesie Dog* (1 serving)
Pretzel sticks (20, small)
Dried apricots (4 halves)
Vanilla Pudding* (1 serving)
Diet Kool-Aid of choice (as desired)

AFTERNOON SNACK

Fried Rice* (1 serving)
Chow mein noodles (2 ounces)
Diet Kool-Aid of choice (as desired)

DINNER

Olé Mexi-Casserole* (1 serving)
Corn and Cauliflower Mix* (2 servings)
Lime-Applesauce Gelatin* (1 serving)
Chocolate Skim Milk* (1 serving)

EVENING SNACK

Salty Corn Chips* (1 serving)
Johnny C's Spicy Sauce* (as desired)
Orange juice (½ cup)

DIET PLAN C

DAY 9

BREAKFAST

Orange juice (½ cup)
Cinnamon French Toast* (2 slices) **with diet margarine** (2 teaspoons)
Special Syrup* (as desired)
Orange-Raisin Spread* (2 servings)
Cornflakes (¾ cup)
Skim milk (1 cup)

LUNCH

Sandwich: Pizza Burger* (1 serving)
Salty Corn Chips* (1 serving)
Apple (1, medium-sized)
Skim milk (1 cup)

AFTERNOON SNACK

Cheesy Celery* (1 serving)
Wheat Thin crackers (8) **with Johnny C's Spicy Sauce*** (as desired)
Diet soda of choice (as desired)

DINNER

Tomato juice (½ cup)
Beef Stroganoff* (1 serving) **with noodles** (6 ounces)
Cheesy Zucchini* (1 serving)
Skim milk (1 cup)

EVENING SNACK

Pretzel sticks (40, small)
Raw vegetable sticks with All-Purpose French Dressing* (as desired)
Apple juice (½ cup)

DIET PLAN C

DAY 10

BREAKFAST

Grapes (36, large)
Malt-O-Meal (½ cup) **with low-calorie sweetener** (as desired)
Plain doughnut (1, small)
Skim milk (1 cup)

LUNCH

Hot sandwich: Soft Shell Tacos* (1 serving)
Oven Fries* (1 serving)
Raw vegetable sticks (as desired)
Orange (1)
Skim milk (1 cup)

AFTERNOON SNACK

Tomato soup (1 cup) **with hot dog slices** (1 ounce, in soup or on the side)
Oyster crackers (20)
Diet soda of choice (as desired)

DINNER

Olé Toro Chili* (1 serving) **with shredded cheese** (1 ounce)
Chopped onions (as desired)
Pillsbury buttermilk biscuits
Snow peas (1 cup)
Skim milk (1 cup)

EVENING SNACK

Saucy Apple Cake* (2 servings)
Lemonade* (as desired)

DIET PLAN C

DAY 11

BREAKFAST

Orange juice (½ cup)
Biscuits Kalacky* (3)
Diet margarine (2 teaspoons)
Skim milk (1 cup)

LUNCH

Burger King Double Meat Hamburger (1)
Burger King Fries (1 small order)
Diet soda of choice (as desired)

AFTERNOON SNACK

Sandwich: Bologna (1 slice); Rye bread (1 slice); Lettuce, tomato, horseradish, mustard, (as desired)
Pretzel sticks (20, small)
Diet soda of choice (as desired)

DINNER

Vegetable soup (1 cup)
Chicken Cacciatore* (1 serving)
Rice (½ cup)
Diet margarine (2 teaspoons)
Cheesy Zucchini* (1 serving)
Skim milk (8 ounces)

EVENING SNACK

Raisin bagel (1)
Diet margarine (2 teaspoons)
Orange juice (½ cup)

DIET PLAN C

DAY 12

BREAKFAST

Apple juice (1 cup)
Fried bologna (2 slices) **on English muffin** (1)
Rice Krispie Square* (1)
Skim milk (1 cup)

LUNCH

Baked potato: (1, large) topped with Chopped ham (1 ounce), Shredded cheese (1 ounce), Chopped green pepper (as desired), Chopped onions (as desired)
Sour half and half (2 tablespoons)
Popsicle (1)
Skim milk (1 cup)

AFTERNOON SNACK

Chicken noodle soup (1 cup)
Oyster crackers (20)

DINNER

Stuffed Green Peppers* (1 serving)
Mixed vegetables (½ cup)
Lettuce salad (as desired) **with croutons** (2 ounces) **and All-Purpose French Dressing*** (as desired)
Dinner rolls (2)
Skim milk (1 cup)

EVENING SNACK

Saucy Apple Cake* (2 servings)

DIET PLAN C

DAY 13

BREAKFAST

Grape juice (¾ cup)
Chocolate Cream of Wheat (½ cup) **with low-calorie sweetener** (as desired)
Applesauce Muffins* (2)
Vanilla Yogurt* (1 cup)

LUNCH

Chicken noodle soup (1 cup)
Sandwich: Peanut butter (2 tablespoons), Diet jelly (2 teaspoons), Whole wheat bread (2 slices)
Pear-Half Gelatin* (1 serving. See recipe for Fruit Salad Mold*)
Cheesy Celery* (2 servings)
Skim milk (1 cup)

AFTERNOON SNACK

Spaghettios with Meatballs (7 ounces)
Diet Kool-Aid of choice (as desired)

DINNER

Turkey Egg Foo Yung* (2 servings)
Rice and Chinese noodles (2 ounces each)
Soy sauce (2 tablespoons)
Vanilla wafers (5)
Skim milk (1 cup)

EVENING SNACK

Raisin toast (2 slices)
Orange-Raisin Spread* (1 serving)
Tea with low-calorie sweetener (as desired)

DIET PLAN C

DAY 14

BREAKFAST

Cantaloupe (½ small)
Banana Fruity Milk* (1 serving)
Applesauce Muffins* (3)
Diet margarine (2 teaspoons)

LUNCH

Taco Bell Combination Burrito (1)
Orange (1)
Skim milk (1 cup)

AFTERNOON SNACK

Sandwich: Egg (1, medium-sized, use vegetable pan spray), Whole wheat bread (2 slices), Catsup (1 tablespoon)
Raw carrots (as desired)
Diet soda of choice (as desired)

DINNER

Baked Beans* (1½ servings)
Cottage Cheese and Tomato Salad* (2½ servings) **with Low-Cal Thousand Island Dressing*** (1 serving)
Lemon-Lime Gelatin* (as desired)
Skim milk (1 cup)

EVENING SNACK

Float: Diet soda of choice (as desired), Vanilla ice milk (1/2 cup)
Vanilla wafers (5)
Raisins (2 tablespoons)

DIET PLAN D: 2,800 - 3,300 CALORIES

PLAN D INCLUDES:

3 Milk servings	10 Meat servings	15 Bread servings
8 Fruit servings	2 Vegetable servings	6 Fat servings

*BREAKFAST

1 Milk serving	3 Bread servings	2 Fruit servings
1 Fat serving		

LUNCH

4 Meat servings	2 Fruit servings	4 Bread servings
2 Fat servings		

AFTERNOON SNACK

2 Meat servings	2 Bread servings	2 Fruit servings

DINNER

1 Milk serving	4 Meat servings	3 Bread servings
2 Vegetable servings	1 Fat serving	

EVENING SNACK

1 Milk serving	2 Fruit servings	2 Fat servings
1 Bread serving		

A vitamin can be given if desired.

*You may wish to include a food from the meat group at breakfast (an egg, for example). If so, simply borrow a meat serving from lunch, dinner, or snacks.

Using Appendix 1 (page 209), you may choose any food from a group in the amount indicated. Either of the following breakfasts would be appropriate for Plan D.

PATTERN	LUNCH 1	LUNCH 2
1 Milk	Milk (1 cup)	Yogurt (½ cup)
3 Bread		Milk (½ cup)
2 Fruit	Oatmeal (1 cup)	Cereal (¾ cup)
	Toast (1 slice)	English muffin (½)
1 Fat	Orange juice (½)	Orange juice (1 cup)
	Banana (½)	(½ cup)
Free foods	Diet margarine	Diet margarine
	(1 teaspoon)	(1 teaspoon)
	Diet jelly	

BONUS CALORIES

If your child's daily calorie requirement is between 2,800 and 3,100 calories, he will have 300 bonus calories to spend. If your child's daily requirement exceeds 3,100 calories, he will have 500 extra calories to spend.

THE DACHMAN DIET RECIPES

Recipes for the starred items (*) in the following 14-day menu plan can be found in Chapter 9, "The Dachman Diet."

DIET PLAN D

DAY 1

BREAKFAST

Orange juice (½ cup)
Banana (½ small)
Cheerios (¾ cup) **with low-calorie sweetener** (as desired)
Raisin toast (2 slices) **with diet margarine** (2 teaspoons)
Diet jelly (2 teaspoons)
Skim milk (1 cup)

LUNCH

Sandwiches (2): Bologna (4 slices, 95 percent fat free), Rye bread (4 slices), Diet mayonnaise (2 teaspoons), Lettuce and tomato (as desired)
Banana (1)
Diet soda of choice (as desired)

AFTERNOON SNACK

Brick cheese (2 slices)
Apples (2, medium-sized)
Pretzel sticks (60, small)

DINNER

Individual Pizzas* (3 servings) **with pepperoni sausage** (1 ounce. Add to each pizza)
Lettuce and green pepper salad with Low-Cal Thousand Island Dressing* (as desired)
Diet Cola Fizzy* (1 serving)

EVENING SNACK

Applesauce Date Bread (1 slice)
Strawberries (1 cup)
Vanilla ice cream (½ cup)
Orange-Pineapple Milkshake* (1 serving)

DIET PLAN D

DAY 2

BREAKFAST

Mandarin orange slices (½ cup)
Applesauce Muffins* (3) **with diet margarine** (2 teaspoons)
Diet jelly (1 teaspoon)
Strawberry Yogurt* (1 serving)

LUNCH

Hot sandwich: Grilled Cheese Plus* (2 slices cheese)
Apple (1, medium-sized)
Orange juice (½ cup)
Peanuts (10)

AFTERNOON SNACK

Cottage cheese (½ cup) **and Aloha Fruit Salad*** (2 servings)
Rice Krispie Squares* (3)
Vanilla Cola* (as desired)

DINNER

Baked ham (3 ounces)
Baked sweet potato (1, medium-sized)
Brussels sprouts (1 cup)
Diet margarine (2 teaspoons)
Cherry sugar-free gelatin (as desired)
Skim milk (1 cup)

EVENING SNACK

Sandwich: Peanut butter (2 tablespoons), Diet jelly (2 teaspoons),
Whole wheat bread (2 slices)
Orange juice (1 cup)

DIET PLAN D

DAY 3

BREAKFAST

Orange-Pineapple juice (½ cup)
Golden Pancakes* (3)
Blueberries (½ cup) **with Special Syrup*** (as desired)
Skim milk (1 cup)

LUNCH

Hot sandwich: Cheeseburger (1 slice cheese, 3 ounces beef), Bun (1)
Dill pickles (as desired)
Sauteed Mushrooms Or Onions* (2 servings)
Pudding popsicles (2)
Grape juice (½ cup)

AFTERNOON SNACK

Salty Corn Chips* (3 servings)
Lite Line cheese (2 slices, melted over chips)
Johnny C's Spicy Sauce* (as desired)
Orange juice (1 cup)

DINNER

Pork and Beans* (1 serving)
Broccoli (1 cup)
Hot dinner rolls (2) **with diet margarine** (2 teaspoons)
Skim milk (1 cup)

EVENING SNACK

Popcorn-Pretzel Mix* (2 servings)
Banana (1)
Hot Chocolate Skim Milk* (1 cup)

DIET PLAN D

DAY 4

BREAKFAST

Grapefruit (1)
Sandwich: Pork sausage patty (1), English muffin (1)
Cornflakes (¾ cup) **with low-calorie sweetener** (as desired)
Skim milk (1 cup)

LUNCH

Pizza Burgers* (1 serving)
Oven Fries* (2 servings)
Apple (1, medium-sized)
Orange juice (½ cup)

AFTERNOON SNACK

Sandwich: Bologna (1 slice), **Cheese** (1 slice), Whole wheat bread (2 slices)
Angelfood cake (1, 2½-inch wedge)
Grape juice (½ cup)

DINNER

Broiled steak (4 ounces)
Mashed potatoes (1 cup)
Spinach (1 cup)
Corn muffin (1)
Skim milk (1 cup)

EVENING SNACK

Banana Milkshake*
Vanilla wafers (5)

DIET PLAN D

DAY 5

BREAKFAST

Fried Apple Slices* (1 serving)
Cornflakes (¾ cup) **with low-calorie sweetener** (as desired)
Raisin toast (2 slices) **with Orange-Raisin Spread*** (1 serving)
Skim milk (1 cup)

LUNCH

Hot sandwich: Bratwurst (4 ounces); Buns (2); Mustard, onions (as desired)
Fruit cocktail (1 cup) **with whipped topping** (2 tablespoons)
Diet soda of choice (as desired)

AFTERNOON SNACK

Sandwich: Grilled cheddar cheese: Cheese (2 ounces), Whole wheat bread (1 slice)
Dill pickles (as desired)
Biscuits Kalacky* (2 servings)
Orange juice (½ cup)

DINNER

Cornflake Chicken* (1 serving)
Corn on the cob (8 inches long) **with diet margarine** (2 teaspoons)
Ham and Green Beans (2 servings. Variation on Almond Green Beans*)
Tomato and green pepper salad with All-Purpose French Dressing* (as desired)
Skim milk (1 cup)

EVENING SNACK

Alphabet soup (1 cup)
Saltine crackers (6) **with cream cheese** (2 tablespoons)
Canned peaches (2 halves)
Fruity Milk* (1 serving)

DIET PLAN D

DAY 6

BREAKFAST

Orange juice (½ cup)
Crunchy Apple Raisin Oatmeal* (1 serving)
English muffin (1) **with diet margarine** (2 teaspoons)
Diet jelly (2 teaspoons)
Skim milk (1 cup)

LUNCH

Hot sandwich: Cheeseburger (1 slice cheese, 2 ounces beef), Bun (1)
Salty Corn Chips* (2 servings)
Johnny C's Spicy Sauce* (as desired)
Oranges (2, medium-sized)
Eggnog* (1 serving)

AFTERNOON SNACK

Ham and cheese roll on a pickle: Ham, Cheese, Dill pickle (1)
Pretzels (60, small)
Pineapple juice (5 ounces)

DINNER

Ham 'n' Eggs* (2 servings)
Raisin toast (2 slices) **with diet jelly** (2 teaspoons)
Stewed tomatoes (1 cup) **with All-Purpose French Dressing*** (as desired)
Pudding popsicle (1)
Skim milk (1 cup)

EVENING SNACK

Raw vegetable chunks (as desired) **with Onion Dip*** (2 servings)
Saltine crackers (12)
Orange juice (1 cup) **in Diet 7-Up** (½ cup)

DIET PLAN D

DAY 7

BREAKFAST

Breakfast yogurt: Plain yogurt (1 cup), Sunflower seeds (1 tablespoon), Dates (2, chopped), Raisins (2 tablespoons), Vanilla, Low-calorie sweetener (as desired)
Rice Krispie Squares* (3)
Hot tea with lemon (as desired)

LUNCH

Ole Toro Chili* (1 serving. Add 2 slices cheese on top)
Succotash* (1 serving)
Oven Fries* (2 servings)
Popsicles (2)
Diet soda of choice (as desired)

AFTERNOON SNACK

Cottage cheese (½ cup)
Crescent Jamboree* (2 servings)
Bagel (½)
Diet jelly (2 teaspoons)
Diet Kool-Aid of choice (as desired)

DINNER

Tuna Loaf* (1 serving)
Baked potato (1, medium-sized)
Diet margarine (2 teaspoons)
Tomato juice (1 cup)
Lime Opaque Gelatin* (1 serving)

EVENING SNACK

Sandwich: Banana (1, sliced), White bread (2 slices), Diet jelly (2 teaspoons)

DIET PLAN D

DAY 8

BREAKFAST

Grape juice (½ cup)
Eggs (2) **and Ham** (1 ounce)
Cornflakes (¾ cup)
Rye toast (2 slices) **with diet margarine** (2 teaspoons)
Diet jelly (2 teaspoons)
Skim milk (1 cup)

LUNCH

Baked chicken breast (1, medium-sized; about 3 ounces)
Aloha Fruit Salad* (1 serving)
Applesauce Muffins* (3)
Vanilla ice cream (½ cup)
Orange juice (½ cup)

AFTERNOON SNACK

Sandwich: Ham (1 ounce), Cheese (1 ounce), English muffin (1)
Banana (1)
Pretzel sticks (20)
Diet soda of choice (as desired)

DINNER

Sloppy Joes* (1 serving meat, ½ bun)
Corn and Cauliflower Mix* (2 servings) **with diet margarine** (1 teaspoon)
Skim milk (1 cup)

EVENING SNACK

Almost Sherbet* (2 servings)
Raisin toast (2 slices) **with cream cheese** (2 tablespoons)

DIET PLAN D

DAY 9

BREAKFAST

Cinnamon French Toast* (3 slices)
Orange-Raisin Spread* (2 servings)
Special Syrup* (as desired)
Diet margarine (2 teaspoons)
Skim milk (1 cup)

LUNCH

Hot sandwich: Reuben* (1 serving)
Banana split: Banana (1, sliced lengthwise), Vanilla ice milk (1 cup), Tip Top Strawberry Sauce* (1 serving), Whipped cream (2 tablespoons)

AFTERNOON SNACK

Bologna (2 ounces)
Bread (1 slice)
Pretzel sticks (20, small)
Oranges (2, medium-sized)
Diet soda of choice (as desired)

DINNER

Beef Stroganoff* (1½ servings)
Noodles (4 ounces)
Almond Green Beans* (1 cup)
Lime-Applesauce Gelatin* (as desired)
Skim milk (1 cup)

EVENING SNACK

Cheesy Jelly Toast* (2 servings)
Almost Sherbet* (2 servings)

DIET PLAN D

DAY 10

BREAKFAST

Cream of Wheat (½ cup) **with low-calorie sweetener** (as desired)
Doughnut (1, plain)
Grapes (48, small)
Skim milk (1 cup)

LUNCH

Sandwich: Hero (8 inches long; with cold cuts)
Orange juice (1 cup)

AFTERNOON SNACK

Cheddar cheese (2 slices)
Apples (2, medium-sized)
Pretzel sticks (20, small)
Diet soda of choice (as desired)

DINNER

Ole Toro Chili* (1 serving) **with shredded cheese** (1 ounce)
Chopped onions (as desired)
Hot sauce (as desired)
Hard roll (1)
Cooked zucchini (1 cup)

EVENING SNACK

Sandwich: Rye toast (2 slices), Diet jelly (2 teaspoons)
Banana (1, medium-sized)
Peanuts (10)
Skim milk (1 cup)

DIET PLAN D

DAY 11

BREAKFAST

Biscuits Kalacky* (3)
Orange-Pineapple Milkshake* (1 serving)

LUNCH

Hot sandwich: Francheesie Dog* (1 serving)
Oven Fries* (2 servings)
Cheesy Celery* (1 serving)
Peach Opaque Gelatin* (as desired)
Orange juice (1 cup)

AFTERNOON SNACK

Cottage Cheese Cake* (2 servings)
Bagel (1)
Orange-Raisin Spread* (2 servings)
Diet Kool-Aid of choice (as desired)

DINNER

Vegetable soup (1 cup)
Chicken Cacciatore* (1 serving)
Chicken Parsley Rice* (1 serving)
Diet margarine (2 teaspoons)
Cheesy Zucchini* (1 serving)
Skim milk (1 cup)

EVENING SNACK

Peanut Butter Crispy Drops* (1 serving)
Applesauce Muffins* (2) with diet margarine (4 teaspoons)
Dates (4)

DIET PLAN D

DAY 12

BREAKFAST

Orange juice (1 cup)
Sandwich: Fried bologna (2 slices), Whole wheat bread (2 slices)
Corn muffin (1)
Skim milk (1 cup)

LUNCH

McDonald's Quarter Pounder with Cheese (1)
McDonald's French Fries (1 small order)
Diet soda of choice (as desired)

AFTERNOON SNACK

Grape juice (½ cup)
Angel food cake (1, 3-inch wedge)

DINNER

Stuffed Green Peppers* (1 serving)
Mixed vegetables (½ cup)
Lettuce salad (as desired) **with croutons** (¼ cup)
All-Purpose French Dressing* (as desired)
Hot rolls (3) **with diet margarine** (2 teaspoons)
Skim milk (1 cup)

EVENING SNACK

Chicken Noodle Soup* (1 cup)
Saltine crackers (6) **with diet margarine** (2 teaspoons)
Avocado slices (¼ cup)
Lettuce salad with All-Purpose French Dressing*
Skim milk (1 cup)

DIET PLAN D

DAY 13

BREAKFAST

Grapefruit juice (1 cup)
Malt-O-Meal (½ cup) **with low-calorie sweetener** (as desired)
Special Syrup* (as desired)
Applesauce Muffins* (2) **with diet jelly** (2 teaspoons)
Vanilla Yogurt* (1 serving)

LUNCH

Cheesy Macaroni* (2 servings)
Plums (4, small)
Dill pickles (as desired)
Vanilla wafers (10)
Lemonade* (as desired)

AFTERNOON SNACK

Sandwich: Grilled Cheese Plus* (1 double)
Dill pickles (as desired)
Pretzel sticks (10, small)
Orange juice (1 cup)

DINNER

Turkey Egg Foo Yung* (2 servings)
Rice and Chinese noodles (2 ounces each)
Rice Krispie Squares* (2)
Diet soda of choice (as desired)

EVENING SNACK

Banana split: Banana (1), Vanilla ice cream (½ cup), Tip Top Strawberry Sauce* (1 serving)
Vanilla wafers (5)
Skim milk (1 cup)

DIET PLAN D

DAY 14

BREAKFAST

Grapefruit (½)
Fruity Milk* (1 serving)
Graham crackers (6, 2½-inch squares)
Diet margarine (2 teaspoons)

LUNCH

Minestrone soup (1 cup)
Sandwich: Oven Swiss Steak* (2 servings), Whole wheat bread (2 slices)
Vanilla ice cream (½ cup)
Apple juice (¾ cup)

AFTERNOON SNACK

Sandwich: Ham (1 ounce); Cheese (1 ounce); English muffin (1);
Lettuce, mustard, dill pickles (as desired)
Pretzel sticks (10, small)
Grapes (24, small)
Diet soda of choice (as desired)

DINNER

Ginger Pork Chops* (1 serving)
Baked Beans* (1 serving)
Mashed potatoes (½ cup)
Diet margarine (2 teaspoons)
Skim milk (1 cup)

EVENING SNACK

Chocolate-Coconut Drops* (2 servings)
Skim milk (1 cup)

9

THE DACHMAN DIET RECIPES

GOOD-tasting meals do not have to consist of high-calorie, fat-ridden, unhealthful foods. As a matter of fact, you may find that your child likes the low-calorie versions of some of his favorite foods even better than their high-calorie counterparts.

It wouldn't make sense for me to offer you a hundred pages of recipes in this book, since it is not a cookbook, but because I realize that pleasant-tasting, low-calorie recipes can be of great importance to a dieter, I have included recipes for entrees; vegetables; beverages; salads, dressings, and jellos; appetizers, snacks, and side dishes; breakfast dishes; desserts and sweets; and yogurts and puddings. All the recipes may easily be incorporated into your child's diet plan. Simply look at the serving sizes and portion equivalents included with each recipe to find out where you can fit the recipes into his daily menu. Calorie counts are also given with the recipes to make bonus calorie spending easier to calculate.

Foods that appear with an asterisk in the 14-day menu plans can be found in this chapter.

ENTREES

Grilled Cheese Plus

MAKES 1 SERVING
1 OR 2 MEAT, 2 BREAD
330 CALORIES

2 Slices bread
1 or 2 One-ounce slices sharp American cheese
1 Tomato slice, or dill pickle slice

Top slice of bread with tomato or pickle and cover with 1 or 2 slices of American cheese. Add second slice of bread. Coat skillet with vegetable pan spray. Brown sandwich on both sides over low heat.

Individual Pizzas

MAKES 12 PIZZAS
EACH PIZZA = 1 MEAT, 1 BREAD,
½ VEGETABLE
160 CALORIES

12 Frozen baking powder biscuits
1 Eight-ounce can pizza sauce
1 Teaspoon seasoning (of choice)
½ Teaspoon Tabasco sauce
½ Pound ground beef
½ Cup chopped onion
¼ Cup chopped green pepper
¼ Cup chopped mushrooms
1 Teaspoon salt
4 Ounces mozzarella cheese (low-fat, part skim, sliced)

Preheat oven to 350°. Spray cookie sheet with vegetable pan spray. Flatten out biscuits to resemble pizza dough, ⅛-inch to ¼-inch thick. Mix pizza sauce with Tabasco sauce and seasoning and spread on biscuits. Add meat and raw vegetables. Cover with cheese. Heat 10 to 15 minutes until cheese melts.

Ham 'n' Cheese Roll-Up

MAKES 1 SERVING
2 MEAT
160 CALORIES

1 Slice lunchmeat ham
1 Slice Lite Line American cheese
1 Lettuce leaf

Place ham and cheese on lettuce leaf. Roll and close with a toothpick. (This is great finger food for kids and adults.)

Pork Chow Mein

MAKES 6 SERVINGS
EACH = 2 MEAT, 1 VEGETABLE
190 CALORIES

1 Pound pork chops (boned and sliced into strips)
1 Tablespoon vegetable oil
3 Cups sliced celery (bias cut)
1 Cup sliced onions
2 Four-ounce cans sliced mushrooms
2½ Tablespoons cornstarch
10 Ounces beef broth
¼ Cup soy sauce
1 One-pound can oriental vegetables, (drained)

Brown pork in 1 teaspoon of the oil. Drain excess fat. Cook celery, onions, and mushrooms in 2 teaspoons of the oil 2 or 3 minutes, stirring often, until tender-crisp. Drain excess fat. Stir cornstarch into broth. Combine all ingredients. Mix well. Heat, stirring, until liquid is thickened and pork is completely cooked.

Serving suggestions:
Pork Chow Mein may be served over ½ cup cooked rice (1 bread) or ½ cup chow mein noodles (1 bread, 1 fat). You may substitute chicken or turkey for pork.

Barbecued Ribs or Chicken

MAKES 6 SERVINGS
EACH SERVING = 2 MEAT, 1 FAT,
1 VEGETABLE
230 CALORIES

2 Pounds lean pork spareribs
(or 6 chicken thighs)
½ Teaspoon garlic powder
3 Tablespoons vinegar
1 Eight-ounce can tomato sauce
⅓ Cup chopped onion
1½ Teaspoons chili powder
1 Teaspoon salt
¼ Teaspoon pepper
½ Teaspoon oregano
½ Cup water
½ Teaspoon paprika

For ribs:
Trim excess fat from ribs. Cut into 6 serving portions. Place in baking pan. Combine remaining ingredients. Preheat oven to 350°. Bake uncovered for 2 hours. Remove cover; baste; bake 30 minutes more. Spoon off excess fat before serving.

For chicken:
Use the same directions given for ribs as above except to bake for 1 hour uncovered (3 meat, 1 vegetable, 1 fat).

Sloppy Joes

MAKES 6 SERVINGS
EACH SERVING = 2 MEAT, 2 BREAD,
1 VEGETABLE
320 CALORIES

1 Pound ground turkey
½ Cup chopped green pepper
½ Cup chopped onion
½ Cup chopped celery
1 Eight-ounce can tomato sauce
½ Teaspoon mustard
½ Teaspoon salt
1 Teaspoon Worcestershire sauce
Dash pepper
6 Hamburger buns (about 2 ounces each)

Saute ground turkey, green pepper, onion, and celery. Drain excess fat. Add remaining ingredients. Simmer 10 minutes. Spoon onto hamburger buns, allowing ½ cup per bun.

Chop Suey

MAKES 4 SERVINGS
EACH SERVING = 1 VEGETABLE, 1 MEAT
100 CALORIES

12 Ounces diced round steak
1 Spanish onion (chopped)
1 Cup chopped celery
2 Tablespoons molasses
¼ Cup soy sauce
1 Cup chicken broth
1 Small can bean sprouts
1 Tablespoon cornstarch

Spray skillet with vegetable pan spray. Brown meat cubes. Remove meat and cook onion and celery in skillet until tender. Add molasses, soy sauce, half of the broth, and meat. Cover and simmer over low heat for about 45 minutes. Add bean sprouts (and more broth if necessary). Save 1 ounce broth and mix with cornstarch. Add as needed to mixture and thicken to taste.

Lasagna

MAKES 12 SERVINGS
EACH SERVING = 3 MEAT, 1 BREAD,
1 FAT, 1 VEGETABLE

360 CALORIES

1 Pound ground beef
1 Large onion (chopped)
1 Tablespoon garlic powder
1 Sixteen-ounce can tomatoes
2 Six-ounce cans tomato paste
2 Teaspoons Italian seasoning
2 Teaspoons oregano
1 Teaspoon salt
8 Ounces lasagna noodles
3 Cups part-skim ricotta cheese
2 Tablespoons parsley flakes
1 Teaspoon paprika
1 Egg (beaten)
1 Pound shredded mozzarella cheese
½ Cup grated Parmesan cheese

Brown beef with onion and garlic. Drain fat. Add tomatoes, tomato paste, and seasonings. Simmer uncovered 30 minutes, stirring occasionally. Cook lasagna noodles according to package directions. Mix ricotta cheese, parsley flakes, and eggs. In a 9-inch by 12-inch pan, layer noodles, meat mixture, cheese mixture, and mozzarella cheese. Repeat until all ingredients are used. Top with Parmesan cheese. Bake 1 hour at 350°.

Cornflake Chicken

MAKES 6 SERVINGS
2 DRUMSTICKS = 2 MEAT, 1 BREAD

245 CALORIES

6 Chicken drumsticks (or 2 chicken
breasts, halved, each = 3 meat, 1 bread)
⅓ Cup evaporated milk
¼ Cup cornflake crumbs
½ Teaspoon salt
¼ Teaspoon pepper
½ Teaspoon poultry seasoning

Preheat oven to 350°. Wash chicken. Dip in milk and roll in crumbs.
Sprinkle with seasonings. Arrange in a baking pan sprayed with vegetable pan spray. Bake uncovered 45 minutes or until done.

Ham Hash

MAKES 4 SERVINGS
EACH SERVING = ½ MILK, 2 MEAT,
½ BREAD

240 CALORIES

¾ Cup ground ham
½ Cup kernel corn
½ Cup cooked rice
½ Cup chopped onion
½ Cup chopped celery
1 Teaspoon seasoned salt
¼ Teaspoon Tabasco sauce
1 Teaspoon Worcestershire sauce
½ Cup evaporated skim milk
2 Tablespoons grated cheddar cheese
(about ½ ounce)

Preheat oven to 350°. Lightly mix all ingredients except cheese in
large skillet. Cook on low heat until underside is lightly browned.
Turn into 1½-quart casserole dish that has been sprayed with vegetable pan spray. Top with cheese. Heat for 10 minutes to melt cheese.

Oven Swiss Steak

MAKES 1 SERVING
2 OUNCES = 2 MEAT
160 CALORIES

Round steak cut into serving pieces
Salt and pepper (a dash of each)
3 Carrots (pureed in blender)
1 Small jar sliced mushrooms
1 Teaspoon minced parsley
1 Ten-and-a-half-ounce can pizza sauce
1 Onion (sliced)

Brown round steak in a skillet, seasoning with salt and pepper. Place in a baking dish. Add pureed carrots, mushrooms, and parsley. Cover with onion and pizza sauce. Bake at 275° for 4 hours, or until tender.

Chicken Cacciatore

MAKES 4 SERVINGS
EACH SERVING = 3 MEAT, ½ BREAD,
1 VEGETABLE
280 CALORIES

3 Pounds frying chicken (cut up)
½ Cup chopped mushrooms
½ Cup chopped onion
½ Cup chopped celery
1 Twenty-eight-ounce can tomatoes
½ Teaspoon salt
½ Teaspoon garlic powder
1 Teaspoon parsley flakes
1 Teaspoon Italian seasoning
1 Tablespoon cornstarch
¼ Cup water

Brown pieces of chicken in skillet sprayed with vegetable pan spray. Add mushrooms, onion, celery, tomatoes, salt, and spices. Cover and simmer 1 hour. Mix cornstarch with water and add to skillet, stirring until gravy thickens.

Baked Fish

MAKES 4 SERVINGS
EACH SERVING = 3 MEAT
240 CALORIES

4 Fish fillets (cod, perch, white-fish, etc.)
1 Tablespoon vegetable oil
Salt and pepper (to taste)
½ Medium-sized onion (sliced)
1 Tablespoon fresh parsley (minced)
4 Lemon slices
Parsley

Preheat oven to 450°. Place the four portions of fish in a casserole dish. Brush with oil. Sprinkle with salt and pepper. Put lemon and onion on fish. Cover and bake for 25 to 30 minutes. Sprinkle fish with parsley and serve.

Beef Stroganoff

MAKES 4 SERVINGS
EACH SERVING = 2 MEAT, 1 BREAD, 1 FAT
265 CALORIES

½ Pound beef sirloin (cut into 24 chunks)
2 Tablespoons flour
2 Cups beef bouillon (cooled)
2 Tablespoons catsup
1 Teaspoon garlic powder
1 Teaspoon Worcestershire sauce
¼ Cup yogurt
2 Tablespoons sherry

Spray skillet with vegetable pan spray, and brown meat. Set aside. Stir in flour. Add cold bouillon, garlic, Worcestershire sauce, and catsup. Cook over low heat, stirring constantly until mixture thickens. Add meat. Cook until heated through. Add yogurt and sherry. Heat 1 or 2 minutes until sauce bubbles. (May be served over rice or noodles in a quantity determined by bread allowance for meal.)

Pork and Beans

MAKES 2 SERVINGS
1 CHOP AND ½ CUP BEANS = 4 MEAT,
1 BREAD

390 CALORIES

2 Medium-sized pork chops (3 ounces each, without bone)

1 Cup Campbell's Pork 'n' Beans with Tomato Sauce (remove pork and discard)

2 Tablespoons catsup

1 Teaspoon mustard

1 Teaspoon dehydrated minced onion

1 Teaspoon brown sugar

½ Teaspoon Tabasco sauce (optional)

Brown pork chops in a skillet sprayed with vegetable pan spray. Drain extra fat. Mix remaining ingredients and pour into skillet with chops. Cover and simmer 45 minutes.

Stuffed Green Peppers

MAKES 4 SERVINGS
4 MEAT, 1 VEGETABLE
1 PEPPER = ½ BREAD

370 CALORIES

1 Pound ground turkey or beef

1 Medium-sized onion (chopped)

1 Fifteen-ounce can tomato sauce

1 Teaspoon oregano

2 Teaspoons garlic

1 Teaspoon Tabasco sauce

1 Teaspoon seasoned salt

1 Cup cooked rice

4 Large green peppers

Preheat oven to 350°. Spray skillet with vegetable pan spray. Brown meat and onion over medium heat. Drain excess fat. Stir in seasonings, half of the tomato sauce, and rice. Cut peppers in half and remove insides. Stuff each half with about 3 ounces of meat mixture. Place peppers in an ungreased pan. Pour remaining sauce over peppers. Cover and bake for 45 minutes. Uncover and bake 15 minutes more.

Reuben Sandwich

MAKES 1 SERVING
2 BREAD, 3 MEAT, 1 FAT
415 CALORIES

1 Tablespoon diet mayonnaise
2 Teaspoons catsup
1 Teaspoon sweet pickle relish
2 Slices rye bread
2 Ounces sliced corned beef
1 One-ounce slice Swiss cheese
1 Ounce sauerkraut

Mix mayonnaise, catsup, and relish. Spread on bread. Arrange other ingredients on bread. Heat until cheese melts.

Ole Toro Chili

MAKES 6 SERVINGS
1-CUP SERVING = 3 MEAT, 1 BREAD
310 CALORIES

1 Pound lean ground beef
½ Red bell pepper (chopped)
1 Cup chopped celery
1 Onion (chopped and divided)
1 Sixteen-ounce can chili or red kidney beans
1 Fifteen-ounce can tomato sauce
½ Teaspoon chili powder
¼ Teaspoon salt
Dash pepper
6 Slices American cheese

Sprinkle frying pan with salt. Brown beef, celery, pepper, and half of onions over medium heat. Drain extra fat. Add beans (do not drain) and tomato sauce. Stir in seasonings. Cover and cook 30 minutes. Uncover and cook a few more minutes to thicken if desired. To serve, sprinkle some raw onion on each serving and lay 1 slice of cheese over it. The cheese will melt from the heat of the chili.

Tuna Loaf

MAKES 4 SERVINGS
EACH SERVING = 4 MEAT, ½ BREAD

350 CALORIES

2 Six-and-a-half-ounce cans tuna fish (in water)

2 Eggs

1 Teaspoon Tabasco sauce

4 Tablespoons barbecue sauce

¼ Cup chopped onion

¼ Cup chopped bell pepper

2 Tablespoons fresh, chopped parsley (or 1 tablespoon parsley flakes)

½ Cup skim milk

6 Soda crackers (crushed)

1 Teaspoon paprika

Salt and pepper (to taste)

TOPPING:

4 Soda crackers (crushed)

4 Teaspoons diet margarine

Preheat oven to 350°. Drain and flake (lightly separate) tuna; add remaining ingredients and mix. Pour into small loaf pan sprayed with vegetable pan spray. Sprinkle crushed crackers on top of loaf; dot with margarine. Bake for 1 hour.

Turkey Egg Foo Yung

MAKES 4 SERVINGS
EACH SERVING = 2 MEAT, 1 FAT,
1 VEGETABLE

235 CALORIES

6 Medium-sized eggs

½ Teaspoon salt

⅓ Cup diced cooked turkey

3 Tablespoons finely chopped celery and onion

1 Cup bean sprouts

3 Tablespoons finely slivered water chestnuts (optional)

⅓ Cup thinly sliced mushrooms

SAUCE:

½ Cup water

1 Tablespoon cornstarch

1 Teaspoon soy sauce

1 Chicken bouillon cube

Beat eggs and salt until sauce is light and fluffy. Combine turkey, celery, bean sprouts, water chestnuts, mushrooms, and onions. Cook until brown. Turn and brown other side. Repeat 3 more times or until turkey is done. Top with egg foo yung sauce. (This is a good recipe to use for Thanksgiving leftovers.)

Francheesie Dog

MAKES 1 SERVING
3 MEAT, 1 FAT, 2 BREAD
415 CALORIES

1 Hot dog
1 Slice Lite Line American cheese
1 Slice bacon
1 Bun

Split hot dog lengthwise so that it is deep enough to insert cheese. (Be careful not to cut in half.) Place cheese and bacon in slit. Bake in 350° oven until cheese is melted and hot dog becomes crisp. Serve hot with mustard if desired.

Ole Mexi-Casserole

MAKES 6 SERVINGS
EACH SERVING = 3 MEAT, 1 BREAD
310 CALORIES

1 Pound ground beef
1 Chopped Onion
½ Chopped Green bell pepper
1 Teaspoon salt
1 Package taco mix
½ Teaspoon paprika
1 Fifteen-ounce can tomato sauce
1½ Cups grated diet Jack cheese
6 Tortillas
2 Tablespoons diet sour cream

In a large teflon frying pan saute meat, onion, and pepper. Add salt, taco mix, paprika, and tomato sauce. Place layer of tortillas, meat, and Jack cheese in a casserole. Repeat until all ingredients have been used. Cover and bake at 350° for 30 minutes. Cut into six wedges and top each wedge with 2 teaspoons sour cream.

Chicken and Broccoli Casserole

MAKES 6 SERVINGS
EACH SERVING = ½ MILK, 2 MEAT, 1
VEGETABLE

230 CALORIES

2 Ten-ounce packages frozen broccoli spears

2 Cups coarsely diced cooked chicken

1 Ten-and-a-half-ounce can cream of mushroom soup

½ Cup skim milk

1 Ounce sherry

1 Tablespoon garlic powder

1 Teaspoon pepper

½ Cup grated cheddar cheese (about 2 ounces)

Paprika

Preheat oven to 375°. Cook broccoli according to package directions. Layer broccoli on the bottom of a 12-inch by 8-inch baking dish that has been sprayed with vegetable pan spray. Spread chicken evenly on top.

Combine soup with milk, sherry, and seasonings; mix until smooth and pour over chicken. Sprinkle with grated cheese and paprika. Bake 30 minutes. Let stand 5 minutes before cutting into 6 portions.

(You may substitute ham or turkey for chicken.)

Pizza Burgers

MAKES 4 SERVINGS
1 BURGER ON BUN = 3 MEAT, 2 BREAD
390 CALORIES

½ Pound ground turkey
4 Ounces shredded mozzarella cheese
1 Small can pizza sauce
4 Hamburger buns

Divide turkey into 4 equal parts and form into patties. Spray skillet with vegetable pan spray. Cook patties over medium heat until browned on both sides. Add 1 to 2 teaspoons of pizza sauce to each patty. Top with mozzarella cheese. Cover and turn heat to low to melt cheese.

Cheesy Macaroni

MAKES 4 SERVINGS
EACH SERVING = 2 MEAT, 1 BREAD,
1 FAT, ½ MILK
320 CALORIES

1 Cup elbow macaroni
1 Small grated onion
1½ Cups grated American cheese
2 Tablespoons diet margarine
1 Tablespoon flour
2 Cups skim milk
½ Teaspoon salt
¼ Teaspoon pepper
Paprika

Preheat oven to 375°. Cook macaroni according to package directions. Spray a 1½-quart casserole dish with vegetable pan spray. Place cooked macaroni, onion, and cheese in dish. Mix well. Melt margarine in small saucepan. Remove from heat and stir in flour. Add cold milk slowly, stirring until smooth. Add salt and pepper. Return pan to heat; cook, stirring constantly, until sauce thickens. Pour over macaroni and mix. Cover. Bake for 30 minutes. Uncover, sprinkle with paprika, and bake 15 minutes longer.

Egg Salad

MAKES 2 SERVINGS
EACH SERVING = 1 MEAT, 1 FAT

115 CALORIES

2 Hard-boiled eggs
1 Tablespoon diet mayonnaise
1 Teaspoon chopped onion
2 Tablespoons chopped celery
1 Teaspoon sweet pickle relish

Shell eggs and chop fine. Mix in remaining ingredients.
Serve alone or with crackers or bread.

Soft Shell Tacos

MAKES 5 SERVINGS
EACH SERVING = 3 MEAT, 2 BREAD

390 CALORIES

10 Ounces ground turkey
1 Package taco seasoning mix
1 Cup water
1 Teaspoon pepper
1 Teaspoon garlic powder
10 Frozen tortilla shells

TOPPINGS:
Shredded lettuce
Diced tomatoes
Chopped onion
Grated Lite Line cheese (3 ounces, about ¾
cup)

Spray skillet with vegetable pan spray. Cook ground turkey over medium heat, stirring until brown and crumbly. Sprinkle with pepper and garlic. Add seasoning mix and water. Stir and bring to a boil. Reduce heat; simmer 10 minutes. To warm tortilla shells, place aluminum foil over a burner on the stove. Separate tortillas and warm, one at a time, over low heat, turning frequently. To serve, place 3 tablespoons meat mixture in shell. Add vegetable toppings as desired and 1 tablespoon grated cheese.

Ginger Pork Chops

MAKES 4 SERVINGS
1 CHOP = 3 MEAT
250 CALORIES

4 Pork chops (¾-inch thick)
1 Four-ounce can tomato sauce
½ Teaspoon salt
2 Teaspoons ground ginger powder
1 Teaspoon garlic powder
1 Green pepper (sliced)

Spray skillet with vegetable pan spray. Season both sides of chops and brown. Remove excess fat. Pour tomato sauce over chops. Cover and simmer 45 minutes. Turn chops once. Slice green pepper and add to chops during last 10 minutes of cooking.

Hamburger Stew

MAKES 8 SERVINGS
EACH SERVING = 2 MEAT, 1 VEGETABLE
180 CALORIES

1 Pound ground beef
1 Onion (chopped)
1 Cup chopped celery
1 Teaspoon salt
¼ Teaspoon pepper
1 Fifteen-ounce can tomato sauce
2 Cups hot water
1 Cube beef bouillon
1 Tablespoon parsley
1 Bay leaf
½ Tablespoon Worcestershire sauce
1 Ten-ounce box frozen mixed vegetables
½ Cup cubed potato
1 Cup noodles (uncooked)

Brown meat, onion, and celery in large saucepan. Add all other ingredients, except noodles. Bring to a boil and simmer 1 hour. Add noodles and simmer 30 minutes more.

Meat Loaf

MAKES 6 SERVINGS
EACH SERVING = 3 MEAT, 1 BREAD,
1 VEGETABLE
335 CALORIES

1½ Pounds ground beef
1 Can vegetable soup
1 Cup fine dry bread crumbs
½ Cup chopped onion
1½ Teaspoons garlic salt
1 Medium-sized bay leaf (crushed)
Dash thyme
Dash marjoram
2 Ounces barbecue sauce

Preheat oven to 350°. Combine all ingredients except barbecue sauce. Pat into 9-inch loaf pan. Spread barbecue sauce over top. Bake for 1 hour.

Peppy Spaghetti Sauce

MAKES 8 HALF-CUP SERVINGS
EACH SERVING = 2 MEAT, 1 VEGETABLE
(WITHOUT NOODLES)
180 CALORIES

1 Pound ground beef
1 Bell pepper (chopped)
1 Small onion (chopped)
½ Cup chopped celery
1 Six-ounce can tomato paste
1 Ten-and-a-half-ounce can pizza sauce
1 Teaspoon paprika
1 Teaspoon salt
1 Teaspoon parsley
½ Teaspoon oregano
⅛ Teaspoon garlic powder
Parmesan cheese

Brown meat, onions, celery, and pepper. Add other ingredients except cheese. Simmer 1 hour. Serve over spaghetti noodles (quantity determined by bread allowance for meal). Sprinkle with Parmesan cheese.

VEGETABLES

Zucchini Fingers

MAKES 4 TO 6 SERVINGS
½ CUP = 1 VEGETABLE
20 CALORIES

1 Small zucchini
½ Teaspoon seasoned salt

Cut zucchini in half, lengthwise. Slice each half 4 to 5 times again, lengthwise. Sprinkle with salt and cook as you would any other raw vegetable. Serve with All-Purpose French Dressing* (page 177).

Ratatouille Royale

MAKES 8 SERVINGS
1 CUP = 2 VEGETABLE, 1 FAT
102 CALORIES

1 Eight-ounce can stewed tomatoes
⅛ Teaspoon thyme
½ Teaspoon salt
¼ Teaspoon garlic powder
½ Bay leaf
1 Medium-sized onion (quartered)
1 Medium-sized green pepper (chopped)
2 Cups eggplant (peeled and chopped)
1 Cup mushrooms (sliced)
1 Cup cut green beans
Pepper (to taste)
3 Tablespoons grated parmesan cheese

Preheat oven to 350°. Sprinkle tomatoes with thyme, garlic, and salt. Let stand. Saute remaining vegetables until barely tender. Add bay leaf. Turn into 1 ½-quart casserole dish. Add tomato mixture. Sprinkle with pepper and cheese. Bake, covered, for 30 minutes.

Almond Green Beans

MAKES 2 ½ SERVINGS
½ CUP = 1 FAT, 1 VEGETABLE
50 CALORIES

1 Ten-ounce package frozen green beans
18 Whole almonds
1 Teaspoon oregano
½ Teaspoon salt

Chop almonds in a blender or food processor. Mix all ingredients. Heat through according to directions on package.

Corn Casserole

MAKES 8 SERVINGS
½ CUP = 1 MILK, 1 BREAD, ½ FAT
135 CALORIES

6 Tablespoons dry milk powder
1 Ten-ounce package frozen kernel corn
1 Eight-ounce can cream-style corn
1 Cup skim milk
1 Egg (beaten)
1 Cup cornflake crumbs
2 Tablespoons chopped red bell pepper
¼ Cup onion
½ Teaspoon salt
¼ Teaspoon each, ginger and paprika
Dash of red pepper
2 Teaspoons diet margarine

Preheat oven to 350°. Thaw corn. Combine corn and milk. Stir in egg and milk powder. Add cornflake crumbs, red bell pepper, onion, salt, and pepper. Mix well. Pour into one-quart baking dish sprayed with vegetable pan spray. Dot mixture with margarine and sprinkle with paprika. Bake 45 minutes.

Sauteed Mushrooms or Onions

MAKES 1 SERVING
1 FAT
35 CALORIES

3 Ounces sliced mushrooms or onions

2 Teaspoons diet margarine

1 Teaspoon garlic salt

Spray skillet with vegetable pan spray. Melt margarine over medium heat. Add vegetables. Stir until cooked to desired softness, adding garlic salt as you stir.

Snappy Bacon Beans

MAKES 4 SERVINGS
½ CUP = 1 VEGETABLE
25 CALORIES

1 Tablespoon imitation bacon bits

1 Sixteen-ounce can sliced or cut green beans

¼ Teaspoon seasoned salt

¼ Teaspoon pepper

1 Tablespoon dehydrated minced onion

Add bacon bits, onions, and seasonings to beans. Cook over medium heat until juice comes to a boil and beans are heated through. (A small can of drained mushrooms may be added if desired.) For Snappy Ham Beans, substitute 2 ounces of cooked chopped ham for bacon in the Snappy Bacon Beans recipe. Each serving counts for 1 vegetable and ½ meat.

Oven Fries

MAKES 3 SERVINGS
1 BREAD, 1 FAT
110 CALORIES

3 Small potatoes (with skins)
1 Tablespoon diet margarine
Salt

Cut raw potatoes lengthwise. Melt margarine in a small pan. Place half of the margarine in small flat baking pan. Arrange potato pieces on margarine. Brush potato pieces with remaining margarine and bake at 375° until tender. Turn often to brown and crisp on all sides. Salt and serve.

Mashed Squash

MAKES 2 ½ SERVINGS
½ CUP = 1 FAT, 1 BREAD
105 CALORIES

1 Ten-ounce package frozen mashed squash
1 Teaspoon vanilla
2 Patties diet margarine
1 Tablespoon cinnamon
1 Teaspoon nutmeg
1 Teaspoon allspice

Cook squash according to package directions. Add rest of ingredients while heating.

Succotash

MAKES 6 SERVINGS
½ CUP = 1 BREAD
80 CALORIES

½ Red bell pepper (chopped)
1 Ten-ounce package frozen whole kernel corn
1 Sixteen-ounce can lima beans (drained)
⅓ Cup dairy sour half-and-half
1 Teaspoon ginger
Salt and pepper (to taste)

Cook corn according to package directions. Place corn in casserole dish. Add other ingredients and mix. Bake at 350° for 30 minutes.

Baked Beans

MAKES 6 SERVINGS
¾ CUP = 1 MEAT, 2 BREAD, 1 VEGETABLE
225 CALORIES

1 Twenty-three-ounce can pork and beans
¼ Teaspoon salt
2 Tablespoons dark molasses
1½ Teaspoons mustard
4 Slices bacon (cut in half)
1 Medium-sized onion (chopped)
½ Cup catsup
¼ Cup brown sugar

Mix all ingredients in one-quart casserole and bake 1 hour at at 350°. Do not cover.

Potato Skins

MAKES 1 SERVING
1 BREAD, 1 FAT
105 CALORIES

2 Medium-sized potatoes
2 Teaspoons diet margarine

Bake potatoes in 350° oven for one hour. Cut in half and scoop out centers. Add ½ teaspoon margarine to each half. If desired, you may add ½ slice of cheese and return to oven until melted. (Add 1 meat serving to your count.)

Cheesy Zucchini

MAKES 8 SERVINGS
½ CUP = 1 MEAT, 1 VEGETABLE, ½ BREAD
150 CALORIES

2 Small zucchini (6 to 8 inches)
½ Teaspoon salt
½ Cup grated Parmesan cheese
¼ Teaspoon pepper
1 Teaspoon oregano
1 Teaspoon garlic powder
2 Tablespoons diet margarine (melted)
2 Ounces cornflake crumbs
Paprika

Cut zucchini into ¼-inch slices and fry in Teflon pan sprayed with vegetable pan spray. Combine remaining ingredients. Mix well. Pour over zucchini and stir slightly. Sprinkle paprika on top. Cover and simmer for 10 minutes.

Corn and Cauliflower Mix

MAKES 4 SERVINGS
½ CUP = 1 VEGETABLE, 1 BREAD
105 CALORIES

1 Eight-ounce package frozen kernel corn
1 Eight-ounce package frozen cauliflower
½ Teaspoon each of salt, pepper and ginger

Measure out 1¼ cups of corn and 2 cups of cauliflower. Mix and heat according to directions on package. Season and serve.

Spicy Carrots

MAKES 6 SERVINGS
½ CUP = ½ FAT, 1 VEGETABLE
60 CALORIES

½ Cup water
½ Teaspoon salt
2½ Cups sliced carrots
1 Can orange diet soda
1 Tablespoon cornstarch
2 Tablespoons diet margarine
1 Teaspoon ginger
½ Cup canned mandarin orange sections

Bring water to a boil. Add carrots; cover and cook until barely tender. Drain liquid into a measuring cup and add enough orange soda to make 1 cup. Remove carrots from pan. Mix liquids with cornstarch. Cook on medium heat, stirring constantly until thickened (about 2 minutes). Add margarine, ginger, salt, carrots, and oranges; heat through.

BEVERAGES

Vanilla Cola

MAKES 1 SERVING

FREE

1 Twelve-ounce Diet Cola

1 Teaspoon vanilla (or other extract)

Mix and serve over ice.

Soda Fizzy

MAKES 1 SERVING

¼ MILK

20 CALORIES

1 Twelve-ounce sugar-free soda (your
child's choice of flavor)

2½ Tablespoons instant nonfat dry milk

Place dry milk in large glass. Slowly pour in soda and stir.

Eggnog

MAKES 1 SERVING

1 MEAT, 1 MILK

170 CALORIES

1 Cup skim milk

1 Raw egg

2 to 3 Teaspoons vanilla or rum extract

½ Teaspoon salt

Nutmeg

Mix egg in a blender until smooth and foamy. Add remaining ingredients (except nutmeg). Pour into glass and sprinkle with nutmeg.

Natural Fruit Soda

MAKES 1 QUART
½ CUP = 1 FRUIT

90 CALORIES

Equal amounts of fruit juice and diet lemon-lime soda (Example: ½ cup orange juice and ½ cup soda)

Slowly pour diet soda over juice. Stir gently to mix. Serve over ice.

Banana Refresher

MAKES 2 SERVINGS
EACH SERVING = 1 MILK, 1 FRUIT

185 CALORIES

1 Cup plain low-fat yogurt

1 Egg

1 Medium-sized banana

½ Cup orange juice

Place all ingredients in a blender and process until well blended.

Fruity Milk

MAKES 3 SERVINGS
¾ CUP = 1 MILK, 1 FRUIT

160 CALORIES

¾ Cup skim milk

¾ Cup fresh strawberries (or any other frozen berries, unsweetened and partially thawed)

1 Teaspoon vanilla

1 Tablespoon nonfat dry milk powder

1 Teaspoon low-calorie sweetener

Place all ingredients in a blender and blend until smooth. (For a flavor change, add 1½ tablespoons cocoa powder and low-calorie sweetner to taste.) You can also substitute; ½ banana, 4 ounces mandarin oranges, or 3 ounces crushed pineapple bits.

Banana Milkshake

MAKES 1 SERVING
¼ MILK, 1 FRUIT

190 CALORIES

1 Small banana
1 Cup skim milk
½ Cup vanilla ice cream
1 Teaspoon vanilla extract
Low-calorie sweetener (as desired)

Blend the ingredients above.

Orange-Pineapple Milkshake

MAKES 1 SERVING
1 MILK, ½ FRUIT

120 CALORIES

½ Cup drained crushed pineapple
(packed in its own juice)
⅔ Cup nonfat dry milk
8 Ounces sugar-free orange soda
2 Ice cubes

Mix all ingredients in blender. (Save the pineapple juice to drink later.) Surprisingly thick and creamy, like an ice cream shake!

Hot Chocolate Skim Milk

MAKES 1 SERVING

90 CALORIES

1 Milk
7 Ounces skim milk
1 Teaspoon unsweetened cocoa powder
2 Teaspoons sugar
½ Teaspoon vanilla or mint extract

Mix cocoa and sugar in glass. Heat milk. Add a small amount to cocoa and stir until smooth. Add the rest of the milk. Add extract. Stir and drink, or refrigerate and save to reheat later.

Orange Slush

MAKES 1 QUART
½ CUP = ¼ MILK, ½ FRUIT

40 CALORIES

1 Can sugar-free orange soda

1½ Cups fresh oranges

Low-calorie sweetener (to equal ⅓ cup sugar)

Cut orange in pieces and put into blender. Blend until pulpy. Place other ingredients in blender and beat until smooth. Pour into freezer container and freeze until solid. Strawberry or raspberry diet soda and fresh strawberries or raspberries may be substituted.

Lemonade

MAKES 1 ½ QUARTS

FREE

2 Lemons

1 ½ Quarts water

5 Packets low-calorie sweetener

2 Chopped lemon rinds

Lemon juice (optional)

Squeeze lemons. Slice rinds into pieces (about 8 per lemon). Mix lemon juice, rinds, water, and sweetener. Refrigerate for one hour before serving. Add lemon juice, if desired, in teaspoon increments. Mix.

SALADS, DRESSINGS, AND GELATINS

Lime-Applesauce Gelatin

MAKES 4 SERVINGS
¾ CUP = 1 FRUIT
65 CALORIES

1 Package sugar-free lime gelatin
1 Cup unsweetened applesauce
¼ Teaspoon cinnamon

Make gelatin according to package directions. Pour into 4 bowls. When partially thickened, fold 2 ounces of applesauce into each bowl. You may substitute shredded carrots for applesauce.

Coleslaw

MAKES 8 SERVINGS
½ CUP = ½ FAT, 1 VEGETABLE
50 CALORIES

3½ Cups shredded cabbage (about ½ medium-sized cabbage)
¼ Cup shredded carrots
¼ Cup chopped green pepper
2 Tablespoons minced onion
¼ Cup chopped celery
½ Apple (chopped)

DRESSING:
¼ Cup mayonnaise (diet variety)
1 Tablespoon vinegar
2 Teaspoons sugar
½ Teaspoon salt

Combine all vegetables in a large bowl. Mix well and set aside. Mix together mayonnaise, vinegar, sugar, and salt. Refrigerate until ready to serve.

Lemon-Lime Gelatin

MAKES 8 SERVINGS

FREE

1 Package sugar-free lime gelatin
1 Package sugar-free lemon gelatin

Prepare lime gelatin as directed on package. Pour into 8 cups and chill until set. Prepare lemon gelatin. Pour on top of set lime gelatin and refrigerate until set.

Low-Cal Thousand Island Dressing

MAKES 1 ¼ CUPS
1 TABLESPOON = ½ FAT
20 CALORIES

¾ Cup diet mayonnaise
½ Cup tomato juice
1 Teaspoon wine vinegar
2 Tablespoons pickle relish
1 Tablespoon chopped onion
1 Tablespoon chopped green pepper
Low-calorie sweetener (to taste)

Mix all ingredients thoroughly.

Raspberry Gelatin

MAKES 4 SERVINGS
1 CUP = ½ FRUIT
35 CALORIES

1 Package low-calorie raspberry gelatin
1 Cup unsweetened raspberries
1 Cup unsweetened pineapple
2 Teaspoons vanilla

Follow directions on package to dissolve gelatin. Mix in vanilla with cold water. Divide berries and spoon into four bowls. Pour gelatin over berries and refrigerate until set.

Cheesy Celery

MAKES 1 SERVING
1 MEAT
80 CALORIES

Celery sticks
1 Ounce cheese spread

Wash and string celery. Line celery with cheese.
For variety, mix ½ teaspoon Tabasco sauce with cheese.

Cheesy Pear Salad

MAKES 1 SERVING
1 MEAT
80 CALORIES

1 Very ripe pear (peeling optional)
1 One-ounce slice brick cheese
Lettuce leaf

Cut pear in half lengthwise. Remove core. Place on a saucer. Place
cheese slice on pear. Cook on high in microwave for 30 to 40 seconds
or until cheese melts. (Or place in skillet sprayed with vegetable
pan spray on medium heat and cook until cheese melts.) Place on
lettuce. Serve when slightly cooled.

Fruit Salad Mold

MAKES 5 SERVINGS
¾ CUP = 1 FRUIT
65 CALORIES

1½ Cups water-packed fruit cocktail
(or any fresh fruit mixture)
¾ Cup boiling water
1 Tablespoon vanilla
1 Package low-calorie gelatin (any flavor)

Divide fruit into 5 bowls. Make gelatin according to package directions. Mix in vanilla. Spoon equal portion of gelatin into each bowl of
fruit. Stir and refrigerate until set. (You may substitute any fresh fruit
except kiwi, guava, pineapple, figs, or papaya.)

Strawberry Gelatin

MAKES 4 SERVINGS
1 CUP = ½ FRUIT
35 CALORIES

1 Package low-calorie strawberry gelatin
1½ Cups unsweetened strawberries
1 Medium-sized banana
1 Teaspoon vanilla
1 Teaspoon banana extract

Follow directions for Raspberry Gelatin, the previous entry.

Aloha Fruit Salad

MAKES 2 SERVINGS
½ CUP = 1 FRUIT
65 CALORIES

4 Strawberries (halved)
4 Ounces unsweetened pineapple chunks (drained)
½ Banana (sliced)
2 Tablespoons Cool Whip

Mix strawberries, pineapple, banana, and Cool Whip. Place in ice cream dishes and serve.

Opaque Gelatin

MAKES 5 SERVINGS
¾ CUP = 1 MILK
90 CALORIES

¾ Cup boiling water
1 Packet sugar-free gelatin (any flavor)
12½ Tablespoons dry skim milk powder
½ Cup cold water
Ice cubes
8 Ounces plain yogurt

Place boiling water, gelatin, and milk powder into a blender and blend until dissolved. Mix ice cubes and water to make 1 cup. Add to gelatin and stir until dissolved. Fold in yogurt. Refrigerate until set.

Cottage Cheese and Tomato Salad

MAKES 1 SERVING
1 MEAT
80 CALORIES

¼ Cup low-fat cottage cheese
¼ Teaspoon instant minced onion
¼ Teaspoon parsley flakes
1 Lettuce leaf
1 Ripe tomato (quartered)

Reconstitute onions in 1 teaspoon water or tomato juice. Mix onions and parsley into cottage cheese. Spoon cottage cheese onto lettuce leaf and garnish with tomatoes. Serve with All-Purpose French Dressing* (below).

All-Purpose French Dressing

MAKES 6 SERVINGS
FREE

½ Cup canned tomatoes
2 Tablespoons lemon juice or vinegar
1 Tablespoon chopped onion
1 Tablespoon chopped green pepper
¼ Teaspoon salt
⅛ Teaspoon black pepper

Combine all ingredients in blender.Blend about 10 seconds. Cover and shake well before using.

APPETIZERS, SNACKS, AND SIDE DISHES

Creamy Tomato Soup

MAKES 5 SERVINGS
EACH SERVINGS = ½ BREAD, ½ FAT
55 CALORIES

1 Can condensed tomato soup
1 Teaspoon diet margarine

Make soup according to package directions. Top each 4-ounce serving with a pat of margarine. Serve.

Stuffing

MAKES 6 SERVINGS
EACH SERVING = 1 VEGETABLE, 1 BREAD, ½ FAT

115 CALORIES

2 Ounces ground pork sausage
8 Slices day-old or toasted white bread
½ Apple (chopped)
¼ Cup chopped onion
½ Cup chopped celery
½ Teaspoon salt
¼ Teaspoon pepper
½ to ¾ Cup chicken broth
2 Teaspoons poultry seasoning

Fry pork sausage in skillet. Drain excess fat and remove meat. Cook onion, apple, and celery. Add seasonings. Tear bread into bite-size pieces and place in a bowl. Add cooked mixture to bread. Mix. Add broth to moisten.

Creamy Soup

MAKES 1 SERVING
½ MILK, ½ BREAD
80 CALORIES

1 Can condensed soup (10½ ounces, any flavor)
10½ Ounces skim milk

Follow directions on can, substituting skim milk for milk.

Oniony Noodles

MAKES 1 SERVING
4 OUNCES = 1 BREAD, 1 FAT
105 CALORIES

4 Ounces noodles (any type)
¼ Teaspoon dehydrated minced onion
2 Teaspoons diet margarine

Cook noodles as per package directions. Measure out a 4-ounce portion. Mix with onion and margarine. Serve.

Salty Corn Chips

MAKES 8 SERVINGS
1 SERVING (8 PIECES)= 1 BREAD
70 CALORIES

1 Package unsalted corn tortillas
Seasoned salt

Cut each tortilla into 8 pie-shaped wedges. Spread the pieces on a cookie sheet and sprinkle lightly with seasoned salt. Bake at 400° for about 8 minutes. Remove from oven and, with tongs or a pancake turner, turn each one over. Bake for 3 to 4 more minutes.

Cheesy Jelly Toast

MAKES 1 SERVING
1 BREAD, 1 FAT

115 CALORIES

1 Slice bread (toasted)
2 Teaspoons cream cheese
2 Teaspoons diet jelly

Let cream cheese soften. Spread layer of cheese on toast, then layer of jelly. Serve.

Fried Rice

MAKES 1 SERVING
1 BREAD, 1 FAT

150 CALORIES

1 Slice bologna (chopped)
1 Stick celery (chopped)
½ Small onion (chopped)
1 Cabbage leaf (chopped)
2 Teaspoons soy sauce (or to taste)
½ Teaspoon garlic powder
½ Cup cooked rice

Spray skillet with vegetable pan spray and fry bologna. Add vegetables, sprinkle with garlic powder, and cook on medium high heat until tender. Add rice, Stir well and cook until heated through. Remove from heat and mix in soy sauce.

Italian Loaf Bread

MAKES 24 SERVINGS
1 SLICE = 1 BREAD 1 FAT
115 CALORIES

1 Loaf sliced Italian bread
½ Teaspoon garlic powder
1 Cup diet margarine (softened)

In a small bowl mix the softened diet margarine with the garlic powder. Place bread in the center of a piece of aluminum foil that is twice as long as the bread. Spread garlic mixture on the bread. Wrap foil, folding edges to seal tightly. Heat in 325° oven for 15 to 20 minutes.

Deviled Egg

MAKES 1 SERVING
1 MEAT, ½ FAT
180 CALORIES

1 Medium-sized hard-boiled egg
½ Teaspoon diet margarine
1 Teaspoon mayonnaise
¼ Teaspoon mustard

Shell egg and slice in half lengthwise. Remove yolk. Mix remaining ingredients with yolk until smooth. Divide mixture in half and return to egg halves. Sprinkle with paprika and garnish with parsley.

Peanut Crunch Mix

MAKES 1 SERVING
1 BREAD, 1 FAT

105 CALORIES

20 Peanuts (Spanish variety)
½ Cup Cheerios or 20 small pretzel sticks

Mix and serve.

Popcorn-Pretzel Mix

MAKES 1 SERVING
2 BREAD

140 CALORIES

1 Cup popped popcorn
20 Small pretzel sticks

Mix and serve.

Onion Dip

MAKES 1 SERVING
1 FAT

35 CALORIES

2 Ounces diet sour cream
Dehydrated minced onions (to taste)

Mix and serve.

Chicken and Parsley Rice

MAKES 2 SERVINGS
½ CUP = 1 BREAD
70 CALORIES

⅔ Cup water
¾ Teaspoon fat-free chicken broth
1 Teaspoon parsley flakes
⅔ Cup instant rice

Bring water to a boil. Dissolve chicken broth in water. Add parsley. Stir in rice, cover, and remove from heat. Let stand 5 minutes.

Johnny C's Spicy Sauce

MAKES ¾ CUP
FREE

1 Ten-ounce can tomatoes
1 Small onion (finely chopped)
1 Teaspoon oregano
1 Teaspoon chili powder
1 Teaspoon garlic powder
1 Teaspoon Tabasco sauce (optional)

Place tomatoes and juice in a bowl. Chop tomatoes into small chunks. Add onion and seasonings. Serve with raw vegetables. (This is even better after refrigerating overnight.)

Hors D'Oeuvres

MAKES 1 SERVING
1 BREAD, 2 MEAT
230 CALORIES

1 Slice bologna
1 Slice American cheese
Crackers to equal 70 calories
(for example, 6 Saltine crackers = 70
calories)

Cut bologna and cheese into 6 pieces. Place 1 piece of meat and cheese on each cracker. Garnish with parsley.

Paprika White Sauce

MAKES 2 SERVINGS
½ CUP = ½ MILK
45 CALORIES

1 Tablespoon flour
1 Cup skim milk
½ Teaspoon salt
⅛ Teaspoon pepper
¼ Teaspoon paprika

Mix flour in 1 ounce of cold milk to form a pasty liquid. Blend in seasonings. Warm remaining milk. Mix in flour paste, stirring constantly. Remove from heat when sauce thickens.

DESSERTS AND SWEETS

Peanut Butter Crispy Drops

MAKES 8 DROPS
2 DROPS = ½ MEAT, 1 BREAD, 1 FAT
165 CALORIES

¼ Cup peanut butter
¼ Skim milk (divided)
¼ Cup raisins
4 Graham crackers (2 half-inch squares, or ½ cup Rice Krispies)
Dash cinnamon
1 Teaspoon maple extract

Cream peanut butter with 2 tablespoons milk until well blended. Add remaining ingredients. Mix well. Drop on aluminum foil or wax paper in balls about 1 inch in diameter. Place in freezer until ready to serve.

Pretty Pastel Cookies

MAKES 4 DOZEN
2 COOKIES = ¼ MILK
20 CALORIES

4 Egg whites
½ Cup nonfat dry milk
1 Teaspoon vanilla
Low-calorie sweetener (to equal ¼ cup sugar)
Sugar-free fruit-flavored gelatin

With an electric mixer, beat egg whites until very stiff. Add powdered milk and mix on low speed. Add vanilla and sweetener. Drop by teaspoonful on an ungreased cookie sheet. Bake at 275° for 40 to 45 minutes until dry and lightly browned. Remove from oven and sprinkle lightly with different colors of gelatin.

Crescent Jamboree

MAKES 8 SERVINGS
1 COOKIE = 1 BREAD, 1 FRUIT

135 CALORIES

1 Can refrigerated crescent roll
dough

Currant jelly (or pie filling,
or your favorite jam)

Pull dough apart in sections. Spread jelly (1 level tablespoon) on each
triangle. Roll triangles from the wide end. Bake as directed on package.

Applesauce Date Bread

MAKES 16 SLICES
EACH SLICE = 2 BREAD
(OR 1 FRUIT, 1 FAT)

235 CALORIES

1 Egg (slightly beaten)

¾ Cup unsweetened applesauce

½ Cup corn oil

½ Cup brown sugar

8 Dates (chopped)

1 Teaspoon vanilla

1 Cup wheat flour

2 Teaspoons baking powder

½ Teaspoon salt

1½ Teaspoons cinnamon

½ Teaspoon ground cloves

¾ Cup crushed graham crackers

Preheat oven to 350°. Combine first 6 ingredients and mix well. Sift
flour, baking powder, salt, and spices together. Mix into applesauce
mixture. Pour into a 9-inch by 5-inch loaf pan sprayed with vegetable
pan spray. Bake for 1 hour. Cool 10 minutes before removing from pan.
(Tip: Let bread cool for several hours or overnight for easier slicing.)

Chocolate-Coconut Drops

MAKES 6 SERVINGS
EACH SERVING (5 DROPS) = 1 BREAD, 1
FAT, 1 FRUIT (OR 1 BREAD, 2 FAT)

155 CALORIES

2 Ounces baking chocolate

1 Ounce semisweet chocolate bits
(about 65 pieces)

½ Cup shredded coconut

3½ Cups of any unsweetened cereal

Melt chocolate in heavy pan over low heat, stirring occasionally. Add coconut and cereal; stir to coat. Drop by tablespoons onto cookie sheet covered with waxed paper. Chill in refrigerator. Makes 30 mounds. (Once chilled, these may be kept at room temperature.)

Freezer Fudge Bars

MAKES 4 SERVINGS
EACH SERVING = ½ MILK

40 CALORIES

1 Envelope chocolate instant
breakfast drink

¾ Cup skim milk

1 Teaspoon mint extract (optional)

Process ingredients in blender for 30 seconds. Pour mixture into 4 small waxed-paper cups or freezer pop containers. Place popsicle stick in each cup. Freeze.

Cream Cheese Frosting

MAKES 4 SERVINGS
EACH SERVING = 1 FAT

30 CALORIES

6 Tablespoons reduced-calorie
cream cheese

Low-calorie sweetener (to taste)

½ Teaspoon vanilla

1 Teaspoon unsweetened cocoa powder
(optional)

Soften cream cheese by allowing it to sit at room temperature for 20 to
30 minutes. Mix in remaining ingredients.

Strawberry Shortcake

MAKES 1 SERVING
2 BREAD, 1 FRUIT

160 CALORIES

¾ Cup fresh or frozen strawberries
(unsweetened)

2 Tablespoons sugar

1 Tablespoon water

1 Slice angel or sponge cake (about 1 inch
thick)

Wash, drain, and hull strawberries; cut in halves or quarters. Add sugar and water. Refrigerate 2 hours. Serve over cake. Suggested toppings:
2 tablespoons sour cream (1 fat; add 40 calories); 1 tablespoon plain
yogurt (free); 4 ounces vanilla ice cream (1 bread, 2 fat; add 130 calories); or 4 ounces vanilla ice milk (1 bread, 1 fat; add 100 calories).

Tip Top Strawberry Sauce

MAKES 3 CUPS
2 TO 3 TABLESPOONS, FREE 4
TABLESPOONS = 1 FRUIT (or 1 fat)
50 CALORIES

1 Envelope sugar-free strawberry jello
1 Cup fresh strawberries
2½ Cups water (1 cup hot, 1½ cups cold)

Dissolve jello in the hot water, then add cold water. Crush berries with potato masher. Mix together. Keep refrigerated in covered container (lasts about 1 week). Use as topping for treats or mix with skim milk as strawberry milk drink. Substitute blueberries, raspberries, crushed pineapple (unsweetened), or banana if desired.

Rice Krispie Squares

MAKES 16 SERVINGS
EACH SERVING = 1 BREAD
95 CALORIES

¼ Cup butter (½ stick)
2 Cups dates (chopped)
2½ Cups Rice Krispies
½ Teaspoon vanilla

Melt butter in small pan. Add dates and steam, covered, until dates are soft (about 15 minutes). Remove from heat. Add Rice Krispies, vanilla and mix well. Pack into a buttered 9-inch by 9-inch pan. Cool. Cut into squares.

Cottage Cheese Cake

MAKES 12 SLICES
1 SLICE = ½ BREAD, 1 MEAT
115 CALORIES

CRUST:

½ Cup graham cracker crumbs
1 Teaspoon low-calorie sweetener
2 Tablespoons softened diet margarine
½ Teaspoon vanilla

Mix all ingredients and press into a 9-inch springform pan.

FILLING:

2 Packages sugar-free lemon jello
2 Egg whites
¾ Teaspoon salt
Low-calorie sweetener (to taste)
1 Cup evaporated skim milk (chilled)
½ Cup frozen orange juice (unsweetened)
½ Cup water
2 Cups cottage cheese
1 Tablespoon sugar

Dissolve jello in ½ cup hot water. Set aside. Beat egg whites until they peak. Add sugar and salt and beat until peaks are stiff. Set aside. Beat chilled milk until soft peaks form. Pour jello slowly into milk and beat until stiff peaks form. Set aside. Blend orange juice, cheese, salt, and vanilla until smooth. Pour into milk mixture and add egg whites. Gradually fold all ingredients until thoroughly combined. Pour into springform pan. Refrigerate about 4 hours.

Almost Sherbet

MAKES 2 SERVINGS
EACH SERVING = ½ MILK, 1 FRUIT

110 CALORIES

1 Cup plain yogurt

1 Junior-sized baby food jar of any
fruit (without tapioca)

Low-calorie sweetener (to taste)

Mix yogurt and fruit. Pour into a bowl and place in freezer. Stir with a
wire whisk at half-hour intervals. It will be ready to serve in 1 ½ hours.

Pumpkin Pie

MAKES 8 SLICES
1 SLICE = 1 MEAT, 2 FAT
(OR 1 MILK, 2 FAT)

60 CALORIES

1 Sixteen-ounce can unsweetened pumpkin

2 Eggs

½ Cup Sprinkle Sweet

½ Teaspoon salt

½ Teaspoon cinnamon

½ Teaspoon ginger

½ Teaspoon nutmeg

1⅔ Cups skim milk

1 Nine-inch unbaked pie shell
(pinch up edge)

Combine all ingredients. Pour into pie shell. Bake 15 minutes at 425°;
then reduce heat to 350° and bake 45 minutes longer.

Strawberry Ice

MAKES 8 SERVINGS
EACH SERVING = 1 FRUIT
65 CALORIES

¼ Cup sugar
½ Envelope unflavored gelatin
1½ Cups water
1½ Cups fresh strawberries
3 Tablespoons lemon juice

In saucepan, combine sugar and gelatin; stir in 1 cup of the water. Continue heating over medium heat until sugar and gelatin dissolve. Remove from heat and add remaining water, strawberries, and lemon juice. Pour into mixing bowl and freeze until mixture is firm. Beat frozen mixture with electric mixer or in blender until smooth. Pour into 8 custard cups and refreeze until firm. Let stand at room temperature for 10 minutes before serving.

Jelly Drops

MAKES 3 DOZEN COOKIES
1 COOKIE = 1 BREAD, ½ FAT
100 CALORIES

1 Cup diet margarine
1 Cup cottage cheese
2 Cups whole wheat flour
Diet jelly (any flavor)

Preheat oven to 400°. Allow margarine to soften. Mix with cheese. Add flour and mix. Chill at least 1 hour. Roll to a thickness of ⅛ inch. Cut into three dozen squares. Add 2 teaspoons of jelly to each piece and fold in half. Press edges together with fork. Bake 15 to 17 minutes, or until lightly browned.

Saucy Apple Cake

MAKES 18 SLICES
EACH SLICE = 1 BREAD, 1 FAT
(OR 1 BREAD, 1 FRUIT)

140 CALORIES

2 Cups flour
¾ Cup brown sugar substitute
1 Teaspoon baking soda
1 Teaspoon baking powder
1 Teaspoon cinnamon
1 Teaspoon ground cloves
½ Teaspoon salt
¼ Teaspoon nutmeg
½ Cup diet margarine
2 Eggs
1 Teaspoon vanilla
1 Cup unsweetened applesauce
½ cup raisins

Preheat oven to 350° Mix together flour, brown sugar substitute, baking soda, baking powder, cinnamon, cloves, nutmeg, and salt. Cut in margarine until mixture looks like coarse crumbs. Add, in order: eggs, applesauce, vanilla, raisins. Pour into a 9-inch by 5-inch loaf pan and bake for 1 hour. Cool in pan and slice.

BREAKFAST DISHES

Cinnamon French Toast

MAKES 6 SLICES
1 SLICE = 1 BREAD, ½ MEAT
110 CALORIES

2 Eggs (beaten until smooth)
⅛ Teaspoon salt
½ Cup skim milk
6 Slices bread
1 Teaspoon cinnamon
½ Teaspoon vanilla

Spray skillet with vegetable pan spray. Mix eggs, salt, vanilla, and milk. Dip bread quickly in egg mixture to coat. Brown one side in skillet. Sprinkle with cinnamon. Turn; brown second side. Serve immediately. Can be served with ½ cup applesauce or sour half and half, but be sure to include 1 fruit or 1 milk. You may also serve with Special Syrup* (below).

Special Syrup

MAKES ¾ CUP
FREE

1 Can sugar-free cola
½ Teaspoon butter flavoring
½ Teaspoon maple extract
2 Teaspoons cornstarch
Low-calorie sweetener (to equal
2 teaspoons sugar, if desired)

Dissolve the cornstarch in 1 ounce of cold diet cola. Put aside. Combine the rest of the ingredients and bring to a boil. Add cornstarch mixture. Boil until thickened. (Try other diet soda flavors for variety.)

Applesauce Muffins

MAKES 12 MUFFINS
1 MUFFIN = 1 BREAD

70 CALORIES

1 Egg
¼ Teaspoon cinnamon
¼ Teaspoon allspice
¼ Cup raisins
½ Cup applesauce
1 Tablespoon corn oil
Low-calorie sweetener (to equal 1 tablespoon sugar)
½ Cup enriched flour
¼ Cup wheat flour
½ Teaspoon salt
2 Teaspoons baking powder
1 Cup bran flakes

In a large bowl mix the egg, cinnamon, allspice, raisins, applesauce, oil and sweetener. Stir in flour, salt, baking powder, and bran flakes. Blend until moistened. Divide into cupcake pan that has been lined with 12 cupcake papers. Bake at 400° degrees for 20 to 25 minutes.

Ham 'n' Eggs

MAKES 4 SERVINGS
½ CUP = 2 MEAT

170 CALORIES

6 Eggs
½ Cup sliced mushrooms
¼ Cup chopped green pepper
½ Teaspoon salt
½ Teaspoon garlic powder
Dash pepper
½ Cup diced cooked ham (about 2 ounces)
1 Tablespoon olive oil

Beat eggs and seasonings in a bowl. Sauté vegetables in olive oil until soft. Drain excess oil, if any. Add eggs and ham, stirring gently until done. (You may substitute cooked turkey, if desired.)

Crunchy Apple-Raisin Oatmeal

MAKES 1 SERVING
1 FRUIT, 1 BREAD

130 CALORIES

1 Tablespoon raisins
½ Apple (chopped)
1 Teaspoon cinnamon
⅓ Cup quick-cooking oatmeal
¼ Teaspoon salt
⅔ Cup water

Mix first 5 ingredients. Bring water to a boil. Add cereal mixture. Stir and heat for 1 minute.

Biscuits Kalacky

MAKES 10 SERVINGS
1 KALACKY = 1 BREAD, ½ FRUIT
100 CALORIES

1 Can refrigerated biscuit dough
Diet apricot jam
Sugar-free jello
1 Egg

Cut each biscuit in half. Roll in a ball and flatten. Put 1 tablespoon apricot jam in center. Fold over and press edges with a fork. Brush with egg white and sprinkle with sugar-free jello. Bake as directed on package.

Orange-Raisin Spread

MAKES 3 SERVINGS
1 TABLESPOON = 1 FRUIT
65 CALORIES

1 Six-ounce can frozen orange juice
2 Cups raisins

Place frozen orange juice in blender and blend well. Add raisins a little at a time. Place in airtight container and store in refrigerator. May add ½ teaspoon vanilla and/or a pinch of low-calorie sweetener if desired.

Basic One-Egg Omelette

MAKES 1 SERVING
1 MEAT
75 CALORIES

1 Medium-sized egg (separated)
1 Tablespoon water
Dash pepper
Dash salt (optional)

Lightly beat egg yolk with water. Beat egg white in a separate bowl until it forms light peaks. Gently fold egg white into yolk mixture. Pour mixture into nonstick pan or omelette pan sprayed with vegetable pan spray. Cook over medium heat. When the egg mixture sets, gently lift with a spatula and turn. Pour in filling of choice (below) and fold over.

Fillings for omelette:

1. Three tablespoons grated Parmesan cheese and ⅛ teaspoon garlic powder. (Add 1 meat serving).

2. One onion thinly sliced and one cube chicken bouillon. Simmer onion in bouillon and drain. (Add 1 vegetable serving to your count.)

3. One quarter cup steamed, chopped broccoli. (This filling is free.)

Golden Pancakes

MAKES 4 SERVINGS
1 PANCAKE = 1 BREAD, 1 FAT

115 CALORIES

1 Cup wheat flour
¼ Teaspoon salt
2 Teaspoons baking powder
1 Egg
1 Cup skim milk
1 Tablespoon diet margarine
½ Teaspoon nutmeg
1 Teaspoon cinnamon

Measure all ingredients into a mixing bowl. Blend with mixer until smooth. Pour batter in small amounts onto teflon griddle or skillet sprayed with vegetable pan spray. Cook until bubbles form on one side. Flip with a pancake turner and brown on other side.

Cinnamon Toast

MAKES 1 SERVING
2 BREAD, 1 FAT

185 CALORIES

2 Slices bread
2 Teaspoons diet margarine
1 Packet low-calorie sweetener
Cinnamon

Toast bread. Spread 1 teaspoon of margarine on each slice. Sprinkle each with ½ packet of low-calorie sweetener, and add cinnamon to taste.

Fried Apple Slices

MAKES 1 SERVING
1 FRUIT, 1 FAT
105 CALORIES

1 Apple (sliced)
Cinnamon
¼ Teaspoon salt
2 Teaspoons diet margarine
½ Teaspoon brown sugar

Melt margarine in a skillet sprayed with vegetable pan spray. Add all ingredients. Cook over medium heat, stirring constantly until heated through. If more sweetness is desired, mix in a little low-calorie sweetener once apples are completely cooked.

YOGURTS AND PUDDINGS

Maple Custard

MAKES 6 SERVINGS
½ CUP = ½ MILK, ½ MEAT
85 CALORIES

3 Eggs (slightly beaten)
2 Tablespoons sugar
¼ Teaspoon salt
⅛ Teaspoon nutmeg
2 Cups skim milk
½ Teaspoon maple extract
Dash cinnamon

Preheat oven to 325°. Combine eggs, sugar, salt, and nutmeg. Slowly stir in milk and maple extract. Set 6 five-ounce custard cups in shallow pan. Pour hot water in pan to level of about 1 inch. Pour custard into cups. Sprinkle with cinnamon. Bake for 40 minutes or until knife inserted in custard comes out clean.

Strawberry Yogurt

MAKES 1 SERVINGS
1 MILK, 1 FRUIT
160 CALORIES

Make 1 serving of Vanilla Yogurt and add 4 tablespoons of Tip Top Strawberry Sauce* (see dessert section).

Coconut-Rice Pudding

MAKES 8 SERVINGS
EACH SERVING = 1 BREAD, ½ MILK
120 CALORIES

1 Cup skim milk
½ Cup uncooked long grain rice
¼ Cup sugar
½ Teaspoon grated lemon peel
1 Teaspoon vanilla extract
½ Teaspoon almond extract
1 Tablespoon brown sugar
¾ Cup cream-style cottage cheese
¼ Cup shredded coconut

Combine milk and 1½ cups water in top of double boiler; add sugar and rice. Cook covered over boiling water for one hour, stirring often. Uncover and continue cooking until mixture has thickened. Remove from heat and stir in lemon peel and flavorings. Chill thoroughly. Beat cottage cheese and stir into rice mixture. Serve in dessert dishes and sprinkle with shredded coconut.

Lemony Vanilla Pudding

MAKES 4 SERVINGS
EACH SERVING (½ CUP) = 1 MILK
55 CALORIES

2 Cups skim milk
4 Tablespoons instant dry milk powder
1 Teaspoon grated lemon rind
1 Teaspoon vanilla
Liquid sugar substitute (to taste)
Salt

Boil 1¾ cups of the milk with vanilla, lemon peel, pinch of salt, and liquid sugar substitute. Dissolve instant dry milk in the remaining ¼ cup skim milk and add to boiling mixture. After it comes to a boil, turn to low heat and cook for 5 minutes.

Vanilla Yogurt

MAKES 1 SERVING
1 MILK
90 CALORIES

2 Teaspoons dry powdered milk
1 Carton plain yogurt
⅛ Teaspoon vanilla extract
Low-carlorie sweetener (to taste)

Combine all ingredients and serve. (Note: If making yogurt to mix with banana slices, use banana extract in place of vanilla.)

Appendix 1

CREATING YOUR OWN MENUS: A GENERAL FOOD LIST

The tables that follow list foods under each food group as defined by the Dachman Diet. The type of food, equivalent amount of 1 serving, and the number of fat servings (to be deducted from the daily allowance) are listed. The extra fat serving(s) to be deducted applies only to certain foods in the Milk, Breads and Starches, and Meat groups.

Group 1: Milk

TYPE OF FOOD	EQUIVALENT OF 1 SERVING	FAT SERVINGS
Buttermilk (skim)	1 Cup	—
Evaporated skim milk	½ Cup	—
Instant nonfat dry milk	⅓ Cup	—
Skim milk	1 Cup	—
Two-percent milk	1 Cup	1
Yogurt (low-fat, plain)	1 Cup	1
Yogurt (whole-milk, plain)	1 Cup	2
Whole milk	1 Cup	2

Group 2: Vegetables*

TYPE OF FOOD	EQUIVALENT OF 1 SERVING
Asparagus	½ Cup
Bean sprouts	½ Cup
Beets	½ Cup
Broccoli	½ Cup
Brussels sprouts	½ Cup
Cabbage	½ Cup
Carrots	½ Cup
Cauliflower	½ Cup
Celery (cooked)	½ Cup
Cucumbers	½ Cup
Eggplant	½ Cup
Green peppers	½ Cup
Greens:	
Beet	½ Cup
Chard	½ Cup
Collard	½ Cup
Dandelion	½ Cup
Kale	½ Cup
Mustard	½ Cup
Spinach	½ Cup
Turnip	½ Cup
Mushrooms	½ Cup
Okra	½ Cup
Onions	½ Cup
Peppers (cooked)	½ Cup
Rhubarb	½ Cup
Rutabaga	½ Cup
Sauerkraut	½ Cup
String Beans	½ Cup
Summer Squash	½ Cup
Tomatoes:	
Whole	½ Cup
Paste	¼ Cup
Sauce	¼ Cup

*Starchy vegetables are listed in Group 3: Breads and Starches.

Group 3: Breads and Starches

TYPE OF FOOD	EQUIVALENT OF 1 SERVING
BREADS:	
Bagel	½
Bialy	1
Rye or pumpernickel	1 Slice
Raisin (no icing)	1 Slice
White (including French and Italian)	1 Slice
Whole wheat	1 Slice
Bread crumbs (dry)	3 Tablespoons
Bread sticks	4
Bun (hamburger or hot dog)	½
English muffin	½
Dinner rolls (pan or hard)	½ Large or 1 small
Tortilla	1 (6-inch diameter)
CEREALS:	
Cooked	½ Cup
Grits	½ Cup
Dry or puffed flakes (no sugar coating)	¾ Cup
Bran	½ Cup
Shredded wheat biscuits	1 Large
CRACKERS:	
Animal	8
Graham	2 (2½-inch square)
Matzo	1 (6 inches)
Oyster	20 (½ cup)
Saltine	6
Soda	4 (2½-inch square)
PRETZELS:	
Small sticks	20
Twisted	3

FLOUR:

Grains	2½ Tablespoons
Pastas	½ Cup
Rice (cooked)	½ Cup

SOUPS: 1 Cup

STARCHY VEGETABLES:

Baked beans (no pork)	¼ Cup
Corn (whole kernel)	⅓ Cup or 1 four-inch ear
Dried beans and peas	½ Cup
Lima beans	½ Cup
Mixed vegetables	½ Cup
Peas	½ Cup
Potato (white)	1 Small or ½ cup mashed
Potato (sweet or yams)	¼ Cup
Squash (acorn, butternut, winter)	½ Cup

MISCELLANEOUS:

Cake (no icing):	
Angel	1 (½-inch wedge)
Sponge	1 (½-inch wedge)
Gelatin (sweetened)	½ Cup
Gingersnaps	3
Popcorn (popped)	1 ½ Cups
Vanilla wafers	5

The following foods are higher in fat than the above bread selections. If you include these foods in your meal plan, deduct 1 bread serving plus the indicated number of fat servings.

TYPE OF FOOD	EQUIVALENT OF 1 SERVING	FAT SERVINGS
Baking powder biscuits	1	1
Bread stuffing	⅓ Cup	1
Corn chips	15	2
Doughnuts (plain)	1	1
Ice cream	½ Cup	2
Pancakes	1	1

Potato chips	15	2
Potatoes (French fries)	8	1
Pound cake	½-inch slice	2
Taco shells	2	1
Shortbread cookies	3	1
Waffles	1	1

Group 4: Fats

TYPE OF FOOD	EQUIVALENT OF 1 SERVING
Avocado	⅛ (4-inch diameter)
Bacon	1 Slice
Butter (or margarine)	1 Teaspoon
Creams:	
Half-and-half	3 Tablespoons
Heavy	1 Tablespoon
Light	2 Tablespoons
Sour	2 Tablespoons
Cream cheese	1 Tablespoon
Dressings:	
Blue cheese	2 Teaspoons
French	1 Tablespoon
Italian	1 Tablespoon
Mayonnaise-type	2 Teaspoons
Nuts	5 Small
Oil or cooking fat	1 Teaspoon
Olives	5 Small

Group 5: Meats

TYPE OF FOOD	EQUIVALENT OF 1 SERVING
Cheese (low-fat)	1 Ounce
Cottage Cheese	¼ Cup
Egg	1
Egg whites	2 Large eggs
Fish (fresh or frozen)	1 Ounce

Fish and shellfish:

Clams	5 (or 1 ounce)
Crab	¼ Cup
Lobster	¼ Cup
Mackerel	¼ Cup
Oysters	5 (or 1 ounce)
Canned salmon	¼ Cup
Scallops	5 (or 1 ounce)
Shrimp	5 (or 1 ounce)
Tuna	¼ Cup

Lean meats and poultry

(no skin)   1 Ounce

The following foods are higher in fat. If you use them in your meal plan, deduct 1 meat serving plus the indicated number of fat servings.

TYPE OF FOOD	EQUIVALENT OF 1 SERVING	FAT SERVINGS
Cheese (whole milk: cheddar, Swiss, etc.)	1 Ounce	1
Corned beef	1 Ounce	1
Frankfurters	1 Small	1
Peanut butter	2 Tablespoons	2
Sausage (all types)	1 Ounce	1
Spareribs	1 Ounce	1

Group 6: Fruits

TYPE OF FOOD	EQUIVALENT OF 1 SERVING
Apple	1 Small
Apple juice	⅓ Cup
Applesauce	½ Cup
Apricots (fresh)	2 Medium-sized
Banana	½ Small
Berries (all types)	½ Cup
Cherries	10 Large
Dates	2
Figs	1 Medium-sized

Fruit cocktail	½ Cup
Grapefruit	½ Medium-sized
Grapefruit juice	½ Cup
Grapes	24 Small
Grape juice	¼ Cup
Mango	½ Small
Melon (all types)	1 Cup
Nectarine	1 Small
Orange	1 Small
Orange juice	½ Cup
Papaya	¾ Cup diced
Peach	1 Medium-sized
Pear	1 Small
Pineapple	½ Cup diced
Plums	2 Medium-sized
Prune juice	¼ Cup
Tangerine	1 Medium-sized

Fruit may be fresh, dried, cooked, canned, or frozen without sugar or syrup.
Read labels carefully.

Group 7: Free Foods

Some foods have such a low calorie content that they are considered "freebies" and can be eaten in any amount. These are the foods to count on when you're hungry between meals and snacks, or when a snack just doesn't fill you up enough:

Diet Kool-Aid

Dill pickles

Fat-free broth

Homemade iced tea (w/without lemon or low-calorie sweetener)

Homemade lemonade with low-calorie sweetener*

Johnny C's Spicy Sauce

Lemon or lime juice (up to 2 ounces per day)

Popcorn (cooked in an air popper with salt, garlic salt, or butter buds, *not with butter)*

Raw vegetables with All-Purpose French Dressing*

Seasonings (garlic, pepper, herbs, spices, etc.)
Sugar-free candy
Sugar-free gum
Sugar-free soda
Tea

*Most doctors recommend limiting the use of low-calorie sweeteners to 3 to 4 times a day.

Appendix 2

FAST FOODS:
A FOOD GROUP BREAKDOWN AND
CALORIE COUNT

	SERVINGS				CALORIES
	Bread	Meat	Fat	Vegetable	
ARTHUR TREACHER:					
Three-Piece Dinner	6	4	9	—	1,100
Two-Piece Dinner	5½	2½	8	—	905
BURGER CHEF:					
Hamburger	1½	1	1½	—	250
Cheeseburger	1½	1½	2	—	304
Big Chef	2¾	3	3	—	535
French Fries	1½	—	2	—	187
Milkshake	3	½	1	—	310
BURGER KING:					
Hamburger	2	1½	1	—	290
Hamburger w/Cheese	2	2	1	—	350
Whopper	3½	3	4	—	630
Whopper Jr.	2	1½	2	—	370
Whaler	3	2	4	—	550
French Fries	1½	—	2	—	210

	SERVINGS				CALORIES
	Bread	Meat	Fat	Vegetable	
DAIRY QUEEN:					
Big Brazier Deluxe	2½	3	1	—	470
Big Brazier Hamburger	2½	3	1	—	465
Big Brazier Cheeseburger	2½	4	1	—	550
Brazier Hamburger	2	1	1	—	245
Brazier Cheeseburger	2	2	2	—	320
Brazier Hot Dog	1½	1	2	—	270
Brazier Chili Dog	1½	2	1	—	330
Half-Pounder	2	8	2	—	785
Fish Sandwich	3	2	1	—	395
ICE CREAMS:					
Cone:					
Small	1	—	1	—	110
Medium	2	—	2	—	225
Large	3½	—	2	—	340
Dipped Cone:					
Small	1½	—	1	—	155
Medium	3	—	2	—	305
Large	4	—	4	—	450
Chocolate Malt:					
Small	3	1	1	—	345
Medium	5½	1	3	—	595
Chocolate Sundae:					
Small	2	—	1	—	170
Medium	3½	—	1	—	300
Buster Bar	2½	1	3	—	385
Dilly Bar	1½	—	3	—	240
KENTUCKY FRIED CHICKEN:					
Chicken Pieces:					
Breast	—	3	—	—	240
Rib	1	2	—	—	245
Thigh	1	3	—	—	300
Wing	—	2	—	—	160
Cole Slaw	1	—	1	—	125
Two-Piece Dinner:					
Original	3½	4	1	—	595
Extra Crispy	3	4	3	—	670
Three-Piece Dinner:					
Original	4	6	1	—	830

	SERVINGS			CALORIES
	Bread	Meat	Fat	Vegetable	

	Bread	Meat	Fat	Vegetable	CALORIES
Extra Crispy	5	6	5	—	1,070
Potatoes and Gravy	1	—	—	—	80
LONG JOHN SILVER'S:					
Clams with Batter	3	1	4	—	460
Cole Slaw	½	—	2	1	135
Two-Piece Dinner	6	3	6	—	955
Three-Piece Dinner	7	6	7	—	1,190
MCDONALD'S:					
Hamburger	1½	1	1½	—	260
Cheeseburger	2	2	1	—	306
Quarter Pounder	2	3	1	—	418
Quarter Pounder w/Cheese	2½	3½	2	—	518
Big Mac	3	2	4	—	550
Filet-O-Fish	2½	1½	3	—	402
French Fries	2	—	2	—	211
Chicken McNuggets (6)	1	3	2	—	310
Egg McMuffin	2	2	2	—	352
Pork Sausage	—	1	2½	—	184
Scrambled Eggs	—	1½	1	—	162
Hash Browns	1	—	1	—	130
Hot Cakes (no butter)	4	—	—	—	260
Sundae	2	—	1½	—	216
PIZZA HUT:					
Individual Cheese Pizza					
(thin crust, 3 slices):	8½	6	—	—	1,005
Cheese	3	2	1	1	450
Beef	3	3	—	1	490
Pepperoni	3	2	1	—	425
Pork	3	3	1	1	520
Supreme	3	3	1	—	500
Additional Toppings:					
Anchovies	—	—	1	—	30
Green Peppers	Free	—	—	—	—
Mushrooms	Free	—	—	—	—
Olives	—	—	1	—	45
Onions	—	—	—	1	35

	SERVINGS				CALORIES
	Bread	Meat	Fat	Vegetable	
TACO BELL:					
Bean Burrito	3	1	1	—	345
Beef Burrito	2½	3	1	—	455
Beefy Tostado	1	2	1	1	295
BellBeefer	1	1	1	1	215
BellBeefer w/Cheese	1	2	—	1	275
Burrito Supreme	3	2	2	—	455
Combination Burrito	3	2	1	—	400
Encherito	3	3	—	—	455
Taco	1	1	—	1	190
Tostada	1½	1	—	—	190
WENDY'S:					
Cheeseburger (single)	2	4	1	—	520
Cheeseburger (triple)	2	10	—	—	935
French Fries	3	—	3	—	335
Hamburger (single)	2	3	2	—	450
Hamburger (double)	2	6	—	—	630
Hamburger (triple)	2	8	—	—	775

Index